POSITIVE MENTAL HEALTH OF CANCER PATIENTS : AN IMPACT OF PROGRESSIVE MUSCLE RELAXATION

Sanjay Kumar

CHAPTER I

INTRODUCTION

The term „Cancer" is generally used to portray more than 250 similar kind of diseases (Khatoon, 2012), that are incessant in nature. The commonality pertains to attributes that are dangerous as well as strange developments inside any of the attached tissue, because of abnormalities or deviations in the host. These grow at different timeframe, at an alternate pace and differently in various people. Actually, the term "Cancer" is derived from the Greek word "*Karkinos*", meaning crab. Cancer refers to a generic non-communicable disease, in which there is a growth of malignant (cancerous or neo-plasmas) anomalous and irregular cells (tumour/lump) in some or the part of body. These anomalous cells multiply speedily without any obstruction, and spread very fast to local or distant spots in body to form tumours. If not restricted, these tumors may destruct the indispensable organs, may cause an organ failure, or may prompt discharge or stroke/s; in this manner prompting demise if not controlled medicinally. This is the manner by which disease has turned into an extremely keen concern.

Cancer is the key health hazard around the globe. It is an important medical problem as it affects the health status of loads of populace across the world. Over 1.5 million individuals are diagnosed with cancer each year in U.S.A. Though the cancer prevalence and mortality rate vary widely, on an average, the mortality rate due to cancer is one patient in each 90 seconds. It is assessed that almost 75% of the families can have one member suffering from cancer. It is ranked as the second most fatal disease after heart ailment in the United States. 562,875 patients are estimated to die with cancer every year (Center of Disease Control and Prevention, 2011). Though cancer has been ranked second in causing death but it is at the top in creating fear. 1500 Americans were assessed and 49% had agreed with the given statement, "The word cancer itself scares me" (American Cancer Society, 1980).

In India, cancer has turned out to be a major death cause. India is probably getting more than 17 lakh new patients of cancer and more than 8 lakh patients are expected to die per year by 2020. As per single year data of only 2016, over 1.5 lakh cases of breast cancer were reported. The lungs cancer stands right behind in line, with an estimated 1.14 lakh cases, comprising 83,000 cases in males and 31,000 cases in females. (http://www.carehospitals.com, 2017). Cancer incidence in India has been assessed to be 70-80 per 100,000 populations. The prevalence of cancer has been established between 2 to 2.5 million at any time with more than 800,000 new cases per year while death rate is 5, 50,000 per year. Majority of the cases i.e., 70% are presented in advanced stage that causes poor survival with higher mortality. Approximately 6% of the total deaths in India occur due to cancer. This contributes to 8% of total mortality by cancer. These estimates have also established that around 10, 00, 000 people are detected with cancer each year in India (Khatoon, 2012). Recently, the occurrence of cancer has increased and has been diagnosed in nearly 2 people per minute. As per other estimates more than 7 to 9 lakh new cases along with 3 lakh patients die annually with cancer (Rao, Gupta, & Agarwal, 2002). The principal cancer cities are oral cavity, esophagus, lungs, and stomach amongst males. In females these are the oral cavity, cervix and breast cancers causing deaths (WHO, 1999). 50 % of the total cancer related deaths in India occur due to breast and cervical cancer in women. Similarly 50% of death amongst men account to the lung and oral cancers. Leading five types of cancer causing death are; cancers of pancreas, prostate, lungs, colon and breast (Kochanek, XU, &Murphy, 2011). As already mentioned cancer is a leading cause of death throughout; this accounted for 8.8 million deaths in 2015. The cancer of lungs is a cause of 1.69 million deaths. Other cancers like colorectal cancer, stomach cancer and breast cancer are also very common types causing death that led to 774 000, 754 000 and 571 000 deaths.

According to the group Boston Consulting (http://www.dailyexcelsior.com/cancer-scenario-india/, 2014), some studies have shown that 60 to 80% of cancer cases in India are diagnosed quite late and approximately 60% cancer patients don"t have access to quality cancer treatment. The report further estimates that the economic burden of cancer care treatment is the highest when compared to all other diseases.

The cost of a single hospitalisation exceeds the average of annual per capita expenditure of more than 60% of the hospitalised population. Financing of 40% of cancer hospitalization cases are through sale of assets, borrowing and contribution from relative and friend (Rajpal, Kumar, & Joe, 2018).

Cancer has been mainly divided in four categories

Sarcomas – are the malignant neoplasm of the muscles, connective tissues or bones. Osteosarcoma is the most common bone cancer. Soft tissue sarcomas are developed from soft tissues like fat/s, nerves, muscles, blood vessels, fibrous tissues and the deep skin tissues. Though they are not localized, yet they are generally established in legs or arms. These may also be traced in the head, neck or trunk region, internal organs, as well as in the backside of the abdominal cavity or *retroperitoneum*. Generally the sarcomas are not very common tumors, whereas maximum cancers are a type of tumor called *carcinomas*.

Soft tissue sarcomas generally don"t show any symptoms. Only till the lump grows large enough to be felt, it may go unnoticed. The main symptom is pain. **Explicit symptoms** reveal a particular category of sarcoma. For example, the gastrointestinal system may show hemorrhage in case of tumours, so symptoms like blood in the stool, or a black, tarry appearance may show in the stools.

Risk factors may include age that is generally linked to cancer. The risk of sarcoma has been observed to increase in association to exposure with definite chemicals, which include, vinyl chloride, and phenoxy-acetic herbicides, and dioxins.

Carcinomas are the second type of cancer that usually develops from skin cell or the cells lining organ. The epithelial cells are the reason for it, as they cover the interior and the exterior surfaces of the human body. Carcinomas are the most common type of cancer that accounts for a very large number of cancer patients i.e. approximately 85% of all the adult cancers. These include cancer of the prostrate, breast, colon, lungs, pancreas and skin. One of the six people in USA is affected due to skin cancer, which is the most common and rapidly spreading type of cancer in US (Greenlee, Hill- Harmon, Murray, & Thun, 2001).Carcinomas can occur in several body organs.

Some common categories of carcinoma contain *Basal and Squamous* cell carcinomas (skin cancers), *renal cell carcinoma* (kidney cancer), *Ductal carcinoma* in situandInvasive ductal carcinomas (breast cancers).

Lymphomas are the third type of cancers which are known to develop in the lymphatic system, i.e. in the white blood cells (WBCs) which fight the ailment/s and are a key portion of the immune system of the individual. In lymphoma, irregular lymphocytes start building up in the lymph vessels and lymph nodes, and in other body structures. When such irregular cells proliferate, these may accumulate in one or many lymph nodes or in other such lymph tissues like spleen.

- When such cells multiply and form a mass they are called as a "tumour".
- Often, these tumours surround the tissues and conquer their own space, thereby depriving them of the essential oxygen and the nutrients required for normal functioning and survival.
- Abnormal lymphocytes commute from one lymph node to the other in lymphoma. These may sometimes commute to far-flung body organs through the lymphatic system.
- Though lymphomas remain restricted to the lymph nodes and the other lymphatic tissue, these can also disseminate to the other forms of tissue anywhere inside the body. Lymphoma enlargements outside the lymphatic tissue are called extra-nodal diseases.

Hodgkin and Non-Hodgkin are the two major types of lymphomas:

In **Hodgkin lymphoma** the patients exhibit irregular lymphocytes, called Reed-Sternberg cells, which are formed from the B cells. In **Non-Hodgkin lymphoma** a large cluster of cancers initiate in lymphocytes, which may proliferate slowly or quickly. These may be formed either from B cells or T cells.

The **symptoms of lymphoma** and its signs are very similar to the symptoms of simple illnesses like viral and the common cold that often leads to a delayed diagnosis. The only notable variance is persistence of symptoms even after the viral infection is over. These symptoms characteristically comprise of swelling of lymph nodes without any pain, in the neck and armpits, wherein these nodes are concentrated. Such swellings can also appear in the abdomen and groin, though several patients don"t even experience any such obvious swelling anywhere in the body. The glands when enlarged can put undue pressure on bones, organs, and other body structures causing pain. Nevertheless this pain can be comparable to that of other less serious reasons, again causing a skip of diagnosis. The lymph nodes, along with parts of the immunity's lymphatic system are established across the body, but the inflammation in lymphomas is generally noticeable.

The other symptoms of lymphoma include some swelling in ankle or leg, night fever and moistures, distending or cramping of abdomen, weight loss, loss of appetite, unusual itching, chills, fatigue, pain or altered sensation, loss of appetite, unusual tiredness/lack of energy, breathing problems, stubborn cough, enlarged tonsils and headache. As already mentioned, painful symptoms are usually missing in the primary stages of lymphoma. Actually, painful and inflamed lymph nodes supplemented by some other signs of infection are the signs of dynamic infection. This painless inflammation of the lymph nodes is more common which is accompanied by pain, weakness, paralysis, or otherwise transformed sensations that characteristically arise only when the inflated lymph nodes are pressed against spinal cords or the spinal nerves.

Leukemia is the 4th type of cancer or cancer of blood forming organs, which leads to propagation of white blood cells (WBCs) in blood and the bone marrow. This weakens the immune system. Reduction in regular blood cells makes it tougher for the body to transport oxygen for various tissues, fight infection or even to control the bleeding. Usually, leukemia refers to tumors of the white blood cells. WBCs comprise a very significant part of the immune system. These defend individual body from the attacks by bacteria, viruses or fungi, along with irregular cells or any type of foreign substances. The WBCs cannot function like regular WBCs in leukemia. These also proliferate very rapidly to ultimately outnumber the normal regular cells.

Symptoms of Leukemia:

Due to the immature white blood cells crowding out the platelets in blood, the patient may bleed easily. One may easily get bruises with slower healing and poorer blood clotting. The patient's white blood cells are very significant for combatting infection. When these WBCs or the immune system of patient get suppressed or do not work appropriately, the patients tend to experience frequent infections. In leukemia, the immune system can also start attacking other important „good" cells of body.

With an increased scarcity of good red blood cells, the patient may start suffering from anemia which might result in dyspnea i.e. difficulty in respiration and pallor i.e. a pale skin. These patients may also experience flu-like symptoms, fever, nausea, night sweats or chills, exhaustion, weight loss, and pain in bones. In case of enlargement of spleen or the liver, the patient feels full and eats less, which results in rapid weight loss. Headache is also quite common among these patients, particularly when the cancerous cells have conquered the central nervous system. The problem is that all these symptoms can also be due to other illnesses. Therefore, the diagnosis of leukemia cannot be confirmed before carrying out a proper and appropriate medical expert examination.

Some patients are at a relatively higher risk of developing leukemia due to some suspected or well recognized factor like HIV, benzene, Viruses - HTLV-1 (human T-lymphotropic virus), artificial ionizing radiation, some petrochemicals, alkylating chemotherapeutic drugs consumed in previous treatment of cancers, hair dyes, maternal fetal transmission (rare) and smoking. There is also a sometimes **genetic disposition** sometimes as shown by studies of twins and family history. People with **Down syndrome** and chromosomal abnormalities are also at a relatively higher risk of leukemia.

THE FREQUENT CANCERS

Breast, cervix, lung and prostate cancers are the most frequently occurring cancers which have been discusses below.

Breast cancer begins to develop when some cells of breast start growing out of control. These cells can further invade into many surrounding tissues or may even metastasize to the distant parts of the body. Breast cancer is known to be an entirely women disease, but men can also suffer from this. Breast cancer is a severe disease with latent high mortality and morbidity. It is the most common malignancy in females. E&Y and Ficci Flo released a joint report in 2015. As per this report the breast cancer being 19%, cervix uteri cancer being 14%, the ovarian cancer being 7% contribute to total 40% of all cancers that erupt among women. Kerala, Tamil Nadu and Delhi were reported to have the highest incidence for cancers.

Breast cancer is at the top in the new cases registered in 2016 as per its latest cancer registry in Indian Council of Medical Research and estimated number is 1.5 lakh (over 10% of all cancers). The major somatic concerns of the breast cancer survivors include pain, weariness, sleeplessness, early menopause, loss of fertility, osteoporosis, hair loss, weight gain and mostly the loss of one"s breast. Lymph edema is a common symptom among breast cancer survivors which is very painful. The breast cancer cases in India for the year 2020 are estimated be approximately 123634 in number.

Research has indicated that an amplified negativity of emotions along with psychological distress, particularly anxiety and depression are directly associated with incidence of breast cancer (Ramadas, Qureshi, & Domini, 2015). About a million of new cases of breast cancer are spotted around the world every year (Mahmoud, 2002; Nevidjon & Sawers, 2000). Living with cancer completely changes the life style of these patients (Thomas, 2008). Breast cancer is a stressful experience that negatively affects several dimensions of the patients living with it. Breast cancer poses substantial psychological encounters for the victims of breast cancer. The treatment process itself causes the patients to face issues like pain, altered structure, less satisfied sexual life, psychological sufferings, impaired social life and lymphedema (Enache, 2012; Sen & Aydiner, 2011; Yildiz & Karayurt, 2011). These factors escalate the level of anxiety while dipping the levels of comfort for the breast cancer patients (Aydogan, Doganer, & Borazan et al., 2012; Inan & Ustun, 2013; Kelleci, Aydin, & Sabanciogullari et al., 2009).

Cervical cancer initiates in the cells lining the cervix, that is, the lower part of the uterus or uterine cervix. Fetus is well known to grow in the uterus. Cervix is the connection between uterus and vagina. Transformation zone is the place where both kinds of cells meet together and its placement changes continuously with the age and delivery of the children. This zone is the susceptible zone for cancer. Cervix cancer never erupts suddenly. There are always some pre-cancerous changes and it is not even necessary that everyone having pre-cancerous changes will definitely develop the cervix cancer. Usually it takes quite many years to develop the cervical cancer, yet sometimes it might take less than one year. Therefore, treating all cervical pre-cancers can be preventive.

No symptoms are generally seen in the early stages. Later symptoms generally include some pain in pelvis or pain during sexual intercourse or some abnormal vaginal bleeding. While blood loss after an intercourse may not be intense, yet it is usually indicative of the presence of cervical cancer. Though not necessarily correlated, Human papillomavirus (HPV) infection seems to be involved in more than 90% of the cases. Most of the individuals with HPV infection do not result in cervical cancer. A weak immune system, consumption of birth control pills, smoking, beginning to have sex at an early age or having multiple sexual partners, the other risk factors though less important. The cervical cancer develops typically from precancerous changes over 10 to 20 years. Majority of the cervical cancer cases, almost 90%, are squamous cell carcinomas, while 10% are adenocarcinoma, and a very minor number is the other types. Cervical screening is followed by a biopsy for diagnosis. Medical imaging is necessary to find the extent of its spread. Registries from Mumbai, Delhi and Bangalore have reported the breast cancer to be most profound among females, while cervix cancer is the leading cancer followed by breast cancer as per the rest of registries.

An estimated 122,844 women with cervical cancer are detected, while 67,477 die from the disease every year in India. Around 432.2 million women aged 15 years and older in India are at the risk of developing this cancer. Cervix cancer is ranked as the second most common cancer amongst the women at 15-44 years of age in India. Unfortunately, the age consistent incidence of cervical cancer in India is at its peak at

22 and is also the highest in the South, much higher than 19.2 in Bangladesh, 13 in Sri Lanka, and only 2.8 in Iran.

Worldwide, it is the fourth most prevalent reason for cancer, and also the fourth-most frequent cause of cancer deaths for women. Out of the total cancer death burden, almost 8% of the deaths occurred from cervix cancer in 2012 in the world. Developing countries are more at risk with 70% of cervix cancer burden and low income countries, are under more severe threat of death by cervix cancer. In advanced nations, due to awareness a widespread use of cervical screening programs has drastically cut the cervical cancer rate. Sexual behavior patterns have also been established to cause cancer. Women having multiple sexual accomplices or having a background of frequent STDs, or engaging them in sexual relations at an early age are also at expanded danger of developing cervix cancer (Brownson, Alavanja, & Hock, 1993).

Lung cancers develop due a **wild growth of anomalous cells** in either one or both of the lungs. Lung cancer initiates to develop in the lungs and then spreads to the lymph nodes or other body organs like the brain. Such cancers may spread to the lungs. Such irregular cells do not transmit the routine and required functions of normal lung cells and cannot further develop into healthy lung tissue. Now these abnormal cells can form tumors to obstruct and impede the actions of lungs, i.e. supplying oxygen to the whole body through blood in arteries.

Lung cancer is highly fatal; and thus is leading cause of global cancer mortality. It is also a major healthcare problem in India (Parikh, 2012). National cancer registry Program (NCRP) of India (2012-2014), estimated for an occurrence of 1.45 million cases 2016 and 0.74 million deaths for the year. The rise for 2020 is expected to become 1.73 million cases with 0.88 million deaths.

Being most fatal, the lung cancer accounts for almost 13% of the total new cancer cases and 19% of total worldwide cancer related deaths. Lung cancer accounts for 6.9% of the total new cancer cases in India and about 9.3% of the total cancer related deaths in both sexes. Though the higher mortality occurs in men yet the women do not lag behind in suffering. The highest stated incidences were noted from Mizoram in both the sexes, with an age adjusted rate of 28.3 for males and 28.7 in females per 100,000 populations (Indian Council of Medical Research, 2013). The time leanings of lung cancer have shown a significant and steep rise in metros like in Delhi, Chennai and Bengaluru for both the genders. The geographic region and ethnicity largely influence the occurrence and pattern of lung cancer. The prevalence and pattern of smoking are the most reflecting factors. The overall 5-year survival rate of lung cancer is very bleak, i.e., approximately 15 % in developed countries as compared to only 5% in developing nations. In India, where TB is prevalent, the applicability of the preferred mode of screening tool, i.e. low dose computed tomography or CT is also quite questionable. There is a serious need to develop non-invasive methods/biomarkers for screening of high risk populations as well as for an early diagnosis.

Prostate cancer ranks 2nd as the most common malignancy and is also the 2nd driving reason for cancer mortality in men (American Cancer Society, 2011). Prostate cancer was the most common of a wide range of cancer prevalent amongst men as assessed for its occurrence in hundred and eleven countries in the world in 2008 (International Agency for Research on Cancer and Cancer Research, 2012). Being detected and receiving treatment for prostate malignancy are huge troubling events for most of men (Christopher, Sharpley, & David, 2008). Prostate cancer revealed more regrettable levels of social and affective cancers along with different manifestations such as reduced sleep or insomnia, bowels disorders like unanticipated constipation or diarrhea as compared to all inclusive community (Zenger, Brix, Borowski, Stolzenborg, & Hinz, 2010). Prostate growth is essentially a malady of the elderly men with seventy five percent of cases happening in men having attained 65 years of age or more.

Prostrate malignancy is a treatable disease just in its underlying stage. The prognosis of the „just initiation" prostate malignancy is regularly great even without the medical treatment (Berner, Harvei, & Skjorten, 1999; Gittes, 1991). Unfortunately between 20-40% of prostate diseases are caught at clinically propelled stages (Dickman,

Hakulinen, Luostarinen, Pukkla, Sankila, Soderman, & Teppo, 1999; Maattane, Auvinen, Stenman, Rannikko, Tammela, Aro, Juusela, & Hakama, 1999; Scardino, Beck, & Miles, 1994), when the corrective treatment is not any more conceivable.

Factors influencing the development of cancer

A large portion of the factors procuring such abnormal and deviant growths have already been fixed and are unchangeable. Hereditary variables clearly add to such malignancies. For example a female whose mother or sister has had breast tumour is at almost twice at threat of creating abnormal growth in her breast compared to someone without such a hereditary connection (Claus, Risch, & Thompson, 1993). In any case, just 2 to 5% of breast malignancies are plainly connected to hereditary variables, for example, the presence of breast cancer 1 and 2; thus indicating that numerous other factors may add to the genetics of such malignancy. Elderly and aged people are also more serious threat in light of the fact that the hereditary transformations causing cancer are more likely to manifest with an increased. Notwithstanding, cancer is the second driving reason of mortality for youngsters between ages 1 and 14 years; this isn't just an illness of the old. Accidents are the first and foremost cause for the same.

Ethnicity

Ethnicity is connected with the development of malignant growth or cancer African Americans are under more serious risk than Caucasians (Meyerowitz, Richardson, Husdson, & Leedham, 1998). African Americans are indeed highest in the prevalence of cancer, with most frequent occurrence of lung and prostate cancer among African American men. Latinos and Asian Americans, on the other hand have generally lower rates of cancer. African Americans likely don't have a hereditary inclination to the disease. Most of the studies recommend that these racial differences in occurrence of cancer are due to non- hereditary components like lack of information or knowledge and social factors like poor access to health facilities.

Life styles

Way of life is a solid indicator of the cancer initiation, with some evidences suggesting that 85% of the cancer around the globe could be avoided by changes in individuals' conduct (Brownson, Alavanja, & Hock, 1993). Smoking is also an undeniable one. WHO has assessed that 90% of the oral growth in South East Asia is straightforwardly inferable from the consumption of tobacco and this is the driving reason for oral cavity and lungs malignancy in India (Rao, Gupta, & Agarwal, 2002). Benzopyrene is the concoction in tobacco smoke that prompts lung tumour by damaging the cancer suppressed genes. Indeed, 87% of lung cancer cases are ascribed to „cigarette" smoking only. Smokers are additionally at expanded risk of developing even other types of cancer like cancers of bladder, mouth or pancreas as well as lymphomas and leukemia. The women who smoked were found to be 25% more inclined to die of the breast cancer than the women who had never smoked (Calle, Miracle-McMahill, Thun, & Heath, 1994).

Eating regimen

Diet has been marked as important leading cause of cancers (American Cancer Society, 1980). The women who consume high-fat sustenance like milk, butter and cheese are more likely to suffer from breast cancer (Toniolo, Ribloi, Protta, Charrel, & Coopa, 1989). At the same time the men who have dietary habits of consuming high cholesterol food are twice at risk than those eating low cholesterol foods (Shekelle, Rosspf, & Stemler, 1991). Similarly, individuals consuming more of saturated fats like in red meat are also at a higher risk to develop the cancers of rectum, colon, and prostate (Slattery, Boucher, Cann, Potter, & Ma, 1998). Natural products consumers eating more of fruits, vegetables, green salads or other highly fibrous food are less liable to develop colon and rectum cancers (Slattery et al., 1998; Zhang et al., 1999). Antioxidants are very good and help in preventing the work of carcinogens. Therefore, food containing vitamin A and C bring down the rates of lung and stomach cancers. The diet of the survivors is also important to prevent the relapses. For example, the patients with colon malignancy if consuming meats, fats, refined grains, and sweets tend to relapse individuals with an eating regimen of foods grown from the ground, poultry, and fish (Meyerhardt, Niedzwiecki, Hollis, Saltz, Hu, Mayer, Nelson, Whittom, Hantel, Thoma, & Fuchs, 2007).

Sun exposure has been established to be strong factor causing skin cancer therefore essential to use sunscreens, though people who go for a regular tan do not often use it (Brownson et al., 1993; Koh et al., 2013). *Alcoholism,* particularly its excessive usage has been associated with cancer of throat, pancreas and liver (Heuch, Kvale, Jacobson, & Bjelke, 1983).

Stress, is another serious threat that can cause cancer. Stressful events and experiences, particularly loss of loved ones leads to cancer procurement (McKeena, Zevon, Com & Round, 1999). Studies have revealed that patients having cancer had undergone more stressful and negative events in family. To quote Jacobs and Charles (1980), found that children suffering from cancer were likely to have faced a more challenges and changes in life like injuries or some change in the health of family members before the initiation of such cancers.

Stress is already well established to weaken the immune system. The reduced resistance decreases the ability of body to detect and kill the abnormal cancer cells (Delahanty & Baum, 2001). The stressful events like examination, marital disputes, divorce, and loss of job have been shown to weaken the immune system among human being. At the same time animals are also equally affected by stresses like rotation on a turntable, flashing lights and uncontrollable shocks (in rats), have been shown to reduce the number of WBCs or other immune cells in the blood in rats.

Actually, stress influences the genesis of cancer by prompting the already existing but dormant malignant cells or by debilitating the immune system in such a way that it can no more identify and attack the abnormal cells (Grossrath, Bastisams, Kanazin, Scmidt, & Vetter, 1992).

Researchers have considered **Personality** also to be important factor (Roberts, Newcomb, Trentham-Dietz, & Storer, 1996) many people, including the victims themselves believed. They observed that is caused, at least in part, by personality factors. Personality dimensions, like extraversion, depression and difficulty in expressing emotions have been often associated with cancer development. (Dattore, Shontz, & Coyene, 1980; Persky, Kemthorne Rawson, & Shekelle, 1987; Shaffer, Graves, Swank, & Pearson, 1987). Many people have covered their inner self to appear pleasant and cheerful but they are actually, often passive when exposed to stress. Such people are type C of personality who suppress their negative emotions; and are cancer prone people (McKenna, Zevon, Com, & Rounds, 1999).

Psychiatric and non-psychiatric problems associated with cancer.

Many community based studies have found that there are many comorbid disorders that accompany the active cancers. It is frequently accompanied by both the non-psychiatric and psychiatric issues. Organic mental disorders like presenile dementia usually with depression and the major affective disorders like mood disorders (unipolar and bipolar) are the psychiatric problems that may accompany any type of cancer (Mitchell, Chan, Bhatti, Halton, Grassi, Johansen, & Meader, 2011). Accompanying adjustment disorders include the adjustment disorder with adjustment disorder, depressed mood with mixed emotional features and adjustment disorder with anxious mood (Carlson, Clifford, Groff, Maciejewski, & Bultz, 2009). Anxiety disorders are also very common that include general anxiety disorder, obsessive compulsive disorders (Saniah & Zainal, 2010). Simple phobia along with personality disorder like schizoid personality disorder and dependent personality disorder (Suvisaari, Manderbacka, Keskimäki, Arffman, & Ahlgren-Rimpiläinen, 2017) may also accompany.

Hardly any cancer patients do not face anxiety and depression while suffering from the disease. The signs of depression in cancer patients are tearfulness, sadness, impaired concentration, guilt, hopelessness, suicidal ideation, worthlessness, sleep disturbances and shrunk appetite and sex drive/energy (American Psychiatric Association: DSM-IV-TR, 2000). The accompanying anxiety is also related to the uncertainties related to the treatment, their impacts and possibilities of saving one"s life (Baqutayan, 2012). Feelings of loss of control are very frequent, because cancer patients can neither control the symptoms nor they can stop their treatment.

Though in most of the cases, these issues are temporary and should be deemed as normal responses to a highly traumatic situation, yet they do trouble the individuals and deteriorate the mental health of these patients. Some of the cancer patients reflect these problems to such an intense degree that professional help is required; thus cancer having a double negative effect.

Along with this, the treatment also brings with it many anxieties and routine problems. Cancer is medically treated by surgery, chemotherapy, radiation or a combination of these. Surgery, however small it may be, is always associated with distress. Cancer related surgeries are further related with rejection and fears of receiving less attention and emotional support in future. Post – surgery has been shown to lower level of immunity. The weak immunity may prolong the recovery time and increase the vulnerability to other physiological stress or mental disorders. *Mastectomy*, as treatment of breast cancer along with the removal of adjacent lymph nodes usually crops up chronic weakness and oedema. It also tends to limit the mobility of patients arm. Similarly colostomy i.e. prosthetic replacement of the lower colon has been known to cause a loss of bowel control in patients.

The follow up treatment, is also quite threatening and debilitating, e.g. the radiation and chemotherapy side effects of radiation are severe. Many patients receiving radiation therapy will already anticipate a dreading loss of hair, skin, burns, vomiting, nausea, sterility and fatigue; thus facing fear and anxiety. Most of these conditions actually occur. In India, the patients are hardly ever prepared adequately for chemotherapy or radiation, which might exaggerate their fears and anxieties to heighten the severity of perception of the accompanying side effects; thus reducing the well-being and QOL of cancer patients.

Burish, Meyerowitz, Carey, & Morrow, (1987) have quoted that "At least half of the cancer patients treated with chemotherapy experience some combinations of nausea, vomiting, loss of appetite, sleep problems, hair loss and a feeling of being out of control". Most of the patients enduring chemotherapy suffer from severe nausea and vomiting. Anticipatory nausea and vomiting occurs frequently before the session of chemotherapy to deteriorate the mental health of patients. Administration at the same place, under same circumstances, by the same persons leads to conditioning of patient with a wide variety of stimuli. The vision of hospital staff itself starts causing nausea (Bovbjerg, 1990). Conditioning may occur with the diet taken during chemotherapy (Jacobsen, 1993).Amongst many patients this might lead to hospital anxiety also. The above discussion is indicative of the fact that QOL and well-being are going to definitely reduce in such patients, which were the focus of this study. It is also obvious that such a condition requires a lot of coping on the part of patients which is definitely different from the normal coping required in the normal daily life. The following section deals with all such variable taken in the study.

Positive mental health and cancer

The definition of health given by WHO is quite old and states that "*mental health is a state of complete physical, mental and social well-being and not merely the absence of disease or infirmity*" (WHO, 1948). In other words it was not be wrong to say that it pertains to *"a state of well-being in which the individual realizes his or her own abilities, can cope with the normal stresses of life, can work productively and fruitfully, and is able to make a contribution to his or her community"* (WHO, 2004).

The above definition has orientations which originate from the current development in positive psychology. There has been a time when the emphasis was upon mental illness instead of mental wellness. The distinction between mental health and illness has been well validated empirically. Researchers found modest correlations for the measure of mental illness and psychological well-being (measure of mental wellness) which ranged between -0.40 to -0.55 (Frisch, Cornell, Villanueva, & Retzlaff, 1992; Ryff & Keyes, 1995). Confirmatory factor model is another approach which is statistically very robust, and has shown that the correlation between latent factors of mental health and mental illness in a US sample (n = 3,032) was 0.53; which indicated that only one quarter of the variance between both types of measures was shared (Keyes, 2005). These and other such researches brought a shift paradigm and recovery also caught attention as an important variable of consideration.

Many of the definitions of recovery were proposed (Anthony, 1993; Deegan, 1988; Scottish Recovery Network, 2006) which were based on the experiences of those recovering from mental illness. The most widely-cited definition was proposed by (Anthony, 1993), stating that "*recovery is a deeply personal, unique process of changing one's attitudes, values, feelings, goals, skills, and/or roles. It is a way of living a satisfying, hopeful, and contributing life even within the limitations caused by illness. Recovery involves the development of new meaning and purpose in one's life as one grows beyond the catastrophic effects of mental illness* ". Andresen, Oades, & Caputi (2003) have also expressed in a similar way and write that recovery refers to "*the establishment of a fulfilling, meaningful life and a positive sense of identity founded on hopefulness and self-determination* ".

In this way the emphasis is more on well-being than sickness. This is becoming prevalent around the globe and well-being has become a key focus for developing International policy of mental health in Canada (Mental Health Commission of Canada, 2009) and the United Kingdom (Department of Health, 2009).

This concept is similar to the concept of positive psychology (Seligman, 1995) and the concept of eudemonia. (Frankl, 1984; Maslow,1954; Rogers,1951)were of the similar view. Their emphasis was on what is good in life and what good is needed or required in life. These good experiences include satisfaction, contentment and happiness and flow in the present and in the past hope and optimism for the future. Thinking this way what is important is the „subjective experiences" in life.

When it comes to individual level, this is about the inculcation of positive individual traits, e.g. courage, interpersonal skills, perseverance, forgiveness, the capacity for love and vocation, aesthetic sensibility and originality, high talent, future mindedness, wisdom and spirituality.

On the other hand at the group level, this may be about the civic virtues and the institutions that move individuals toward better citizenship, i.e., developing a sense of nurturance, altruism, responsibility, tolerance, moderation, work ethic and civility.

Such a concept of mental health has been operationalized into mainly three type of well-being i.e. emotional, psychological and social. These have been further divided into 13dimensions (Keyes, 2005; Keyes, 2007). These dimensions (Ryff & Keyes,

1995; Keyes, 1998) are positive affect, avowed quality of life, self-acceptance, personal growth, purpose in life, environmental mastery, autonomy, positive relations with others, social acceptance, social actualization, social contribution, social coherence and social integration.

Following sections deals with various key indicators of positive mental health taken in this study.

Quality of life and cancer

Quality of life (QOL) is an important positive variable that is negatively affected by cancer (Torkzahrani, Rastegari, Khodakarami, Akbarzadeh-Baghian, & Alizadeh, 2013). To understand the concept of quality of life, it is not a very well defined term, though it clearly emphasises components of happiness and satisfaction with life. QOL pertains to evaluation of general well-being of individuals, groups and communities or societies. The term is applicable to a wide range of contexts, e.g., the fields of health care, policies, and even the national and international developments. The concept must not be confused with the idea of living standards, which is primarily based on level of on income and socio economic status. Besides the wealth and employment, the scientific concept of QOL reflect upon the built environment, mental and physical health, recreation, education, leisure time, and also the sense of social belongingness (Gregory, Ron, Partt, Watts, & Whatmore, 2009).

Social and conventional are the two major perspectives that are taken in research on quality of life. Research pertaining to social indicators reflects upon the evaluation of the need of people whereas research on conventional quality of life focuses upon the requirements of people for improving their quality of life (Mukherjee, 1989). Such an approach is known as person centered approach to quality of life. Another vital way to understand the quality of life is health based. As per health based approach, quality of life is considered to be made up of the factors necessary for life sustenance or the factors that enhance or impair the enjoyment in life. This way, healthy life is more important than anything else in life. This approach fails to spot that for majority of people, health is not the end variable which they are aspiring for, but merely a means of achieving the end (O"Boyle, Mcgee, & Joyce, 1994).

However, none can deny that illness and disease lead to serious and debilitating consequences from the physical aspects as these impose restrictions in life while moving in the corridors to happiness. Hope and other types of well-being do get impeded. Accordingly, it is very important to study the health related quality of life of the individuals. Most often the parameters to define quality of life are selected objectively the researchers, with consensus, have focused on all the aspects by considering physical, emotional and the social well-being (Felce & Perry, 1995; Flanagan, 1982; Schipper, Clinch, & Powell, 1990).

As already discussed, cancer has been frequently associated with multiple and serious mental health concerns. This necessitates the investigation of health related quality of life of the cancer patient. Accompanying anxiety and depression lead to poor quality of life and reduce daily activity level of cancer patients (Pedram, Mohammadi, Naziri, & Aeinparast, 2011). "Assessment of disease specific quality of life has gained attention with the realization that the quality of life is differently affected in different diseases" (Jain, Batra, Sharma, & Dahiya, 2011).

Well- Being and cancer

In health cancers, usually both the health and well-being are used interchangeably. Well –being does not refer merely to an absence of disease and sickness. The concept is rather closer to the concerns of mental health, happiness, vitality, energies, self-actualization and the life. Cloninger (2008) has further stressed that "a person cannot feel good (as measured by positive emotions and life satisfaction) without doing good (as measured by maturity of character, and virtuous conduct)". In view of the above, well–being can be described more than it can be defined, though attempts have been made to define it. In their systematic review of the definitions, (Pollard & Lee, 2003), describe well-being as "a complex multifaceted construct that has continued to elude researcher's attempts to define and measure it". It is understood as a dynamic state that should be characterized by attainment of harmony in an individual's needs, abilities, expectations, environmental demands and opportunities.

Well-being has also been defined in terms of physical, social and mental status of an individual that might carry different level of importance for everyone and also exert different impact on each individual (Ebersole & Hess, 1994; Kiefer, 2008). Well-being, when defined within the milieu of health promotion, pertains to the subjective perception and valuation of health which is less concerned with biological functioning and development of positive sense of belongingness through social interaction along with the self-esteem (Nutbeam, 1986). According to Christiansen and Beam (1997), wellbeing may be defined "as a subjective sense of the overall contentment by affective state and life satisfaction". Verma and Verma (1989) have also defined the general wellbeing as "the idiosyncratic sense of happiness, contentment, sense of achievement, satisfaction with life experiences and one"s role in the world of work, utility, belongingness without distress or dissatisfaction and worries etc. in life". Diener has a name in the field of well-being. Diener and Seligman (2004) have stated that "Well-being, which is defined as people"s positive evaluation of their life includes positive emotions engagement, satisfaction and meaning".

Accordingly, subjective well-being is a broad phenomenon of one"s emotional perceptions, evaluations and responses/reactions, domain satisfaction and overall evaluation of contentment in life. Each of the specified construct needs to be understood in its own rights. All these constructs are often found to correlate substantially (Diener, Suh, Lucas, & Smith, 1999). Kahneman and Riis (2005), consider subjective well–being "as a hybrid concept with two ingredients of „experienced" and „evaluated" well–being".

Health Related Quality of Life (HRQOL) is an extremely close concept; in fact very similar. This pertains to the extent to which one"s typical or anticipated physical, emotional and social well-being is affected by a medical condition and/or its treatment (Cella & Tulsky, 1993). The concept of HRQOL is multidimensional. HRQOL as a concept is again challenging to define because it is composed of broad realms of individual"s physical/biological, affective, functional and social subjective experiences. It has become increasingly common for HRQOL of cancer patients has to be included as an important endpoint in large scale clinical trials investigating the effects of anticancer treatment (Victorson, Cella, & Judson, 2008). Assessment and research on HRQOL of cancer patients has good guidance function in specifying on more efficient treatment. Measuring HRQOL provides with information that can be highly useful in understanding the negative effects of disease on daily life of patients. These have been described in second chapter of historical resume.

Emotional well-being has been conceptualized to refer to

1. "A global satisfaction with life, which is based on the individual"s subjective cognitive appraisals about the life in general." (Diener, 1984).
2. "Predominance of positive over the negative effects or the affective balance (happiness)." (Andrews & Withey, 1976; Campbel, Converse, & Rodgers, 1976; Christopher, 1999; Diener, 1984).
3. Diener and Lucas (1999) have stated that "if a person reports that his/her life is satisfying, that he/she is experiencing frequent pleasant affect, that he/she not frequently experiencing the unpleasant affect, he/she said to have high emotional well-being".

Social & family well-being

Social well-being is another construct of mental health (well-being) that has been operationalized by Keyes (1998), who presents following five dimensions of this. These dimensions indicate the extent of healthy and appropriate functioning of individuals in their social world.

- **Social integration** refers to the spread of feeling among people about having something common with others. This „others" refer to those who constitute the social reality of individual, e.g., their neighborhoods. This also refers to the extent to which they feel „belongingness to society" and significant others.
- **Social contribution** pertains to the belief that one „belongs" to society and is its important or significant members. Also one has a faith and trust in individual"s ability that one can make significant contribution to the world.
- **Social coherence** is the perception of quality, planning and maneuver/management of social world. This includes the curiosity and desire to know about one"s social world.

- **Social actualization** refers to the evaluation of prospects or possibilities and course of society. This arises out of the sense that society has enough potential that can be and should be realized through its citizens and organizations or institutions.
- **Social acceptance** is the elucidation of society through the conduct and qualities of the other people. Individuals illustrating social acceptance have trust on others. They believe in kindness and industriousness amongst other people. They possess positive views about human nature and are comfortable with others (Keyes, 1998; Keyes & Shapiro, 2004).

Functional well-being pertains to the individual potential to enable them perform the daily routine tasks and also to manage or effectively carrying out their social roles. It means an individual capacity and ability to carry out routine work does not get limited by any disease or for any other psychological reason.

Fatigue and cancer

Fatigue is hardly ever a binary state: meaning either one has it or does not have it. Everyone experiences fatigue at some or the other time that may vary from mild to prodigious or extraordinary. The concept of fatigue is both vague and highly subjective. Therefore, other descriptors of fatigue need to be seriously considered. These may be named as normal, abnormal, peripheral, or central. *Peripheral* fatigue and *central* fatigue are clearly distinct. Peripheral fatigue pertains to decline in the optimal muscle force or motor output; usually occurring due to persistent and vigorous/strenuous physical work or over exertion. Conversely, central fatigue pertains to a general feeling of weakness, tiredness, sleepiness or languor; which can occur either independently or due to some other underlying pathological or psychological conditions. Normal fatigue has been accepted as a state of general tiredness due to overexertion which is easily ameliorated by taking rest. On the other hand „pathological" or „abnormal" fatigue is characterized by „weariness" that is not related to previous exertions and is often not ameliorated by taking rest. Both peripheral and central fatigue can exist in normal and abnormal states.

Cancer is also known to bring high level of fatigue with it. The National Comprehensive Cancer Network describes cancer-related fatigue "as a subjective, persistent, and distressing sense of either physical, emotional, or cognitive tiredness or a combination of these, not related to recent physical activity and interferes with a patient"s nomal functioning" (Berger, Abernathy, Atkinson, Barsevick, Berger, Cella et al., 2010). Fatigue among cancer patients under treatment is prevalent frequently and is disabling but treatable (Cheville, Shen, Chang, & Basford, 2013). Unfortunately, cancer related fatigue is not being taken into regular account and is underreported and undertreated, where such consideration is imperative to ensure an adequate treatment of cancer. Fatigue is a very common and highly frequent concern amongst the cancer patients as well as the cancer survivor.

For cancer patients fatigue may be understood as a subjective and consistently prolonged or insistent sense of tiredness or exhaustion related to any type of and its treatment which is proportionally more than the recent activity; thereby interfering with the usual functioning (Mock, Atkinson, Barsevick, Cella, Cimprich, Cleeland, Donnelly, Eisenberger, Escalante, Hinds, Jacobsen, Kaldor, Knight, Peterman, Piper, Rugo, Sabbatini, & Stahl, 2000). For cancer patients also it is multidimensional; encompassing physical/somatic, mental and affective aspects. This can be both a presenting symptom of the malignancy and a long-term side effect of the treatment. Up to 30% of the cancer survivors are reported to face a loss of energy even after years of completing their treatment or after recovering from cancer. Cancer related fatigue is often a manifestation of many symptoms as a sum of the direct effect of the tumour and malignancy and the side effects of chemo and radiotherapy along with a reduced nutritional intake or lack of sleep etc. Pain, distress and anemia also occur simultaneously and contribute to fatigue. These factors may be precipitating factors of cancer related fatigue during their cancer treatment amongst women.

Mitchell and Berger (2006) have reported that 78% of cancer patients lived with the distressing symptoms of fatigue. Therefore, fatigue is a vital concern for health care providers. They must conduct research to assess fatigue and understand as its impact with multifaceted problems being faced by patients like weakness, reduced focus and concentration, hypersomnia or insomnia, and heightened or weakened emotional reactivity. Further, it is also important for both the patients and the providers to be able to distinguish depression from the cancer related fatigue. Both providers must also recognize the solid and negative implication of fatigue and depression as factors debilitating for both the patients and care takers. In fact fatigue can reduce resilience and hope thus negatively affecting the coping ways and mechanism.

Hospital anxiety & depression and cancer

The above discussion clearly evincesthat there is very high probability of cancer bringing in anxiety and depression. Multiple evidences have indicated it (Dogar, Azeem, Kiran, Hussain, Mehmood, & Hina, 2009; Farooqi, & Choudhry, 2012; Malekian, Alizadeh, & Ahmadzedeh, 2007; Paul, Musa, & Chungu, 2016; Schwarz, Krauss, Hockel, Meyer, Zenger, & Hinz, 2008; Srivastava, Ansari, Kumar, Shah, Meena, Sevach, & Singh, 2014).

Anxiety pertains to "Anxiety is not the same as fear, which is a response to a real or perceived immediate threat,whereas anxiety is the expectation of future threat" (American Psychiatric Association, 2013). "Anxiety is a feeling of uneasiness and worry, usually generalized and unfocused as an overreaction to a situation that is only subjectively seen as menacing" (Bouras & Holt, 2007). While depression is defined as "Depression (major depressive disorder) is a common and serious medical illness that negatively affects how you feel the way you think and how you act. Fortunately, it is also treatable. Depression causes feelings of sadness and/or a loss of interest in activities once enjoyed. It can lead to a variety of emotional and physical problems and can decrease a person‟s ability to function at work and at home" (American Psychiatric Association, 2013).

The breast cancer is known to be relatively less fatal. Inspite on this, (Arving, Sjoden, Bergh, Hellbom, Johansson, & Glimelius, 2007) have shown that, the breast cancer itself, its diagnosis and the required treatment are all key source of anxiety and depression for breast cancer patients. Actually this kind of anxiety and depression are also associated with many other figures of anxiety within the hospital e.g. surgery has always been associated with fear. In spite of a lot of improvement in technology and improved hospital conditions, surgery is well established to be a source of fear, and anxiety not only for the patients but also for the family members or the other dear ones. Radiation and chemotherapy treatment (Saniah, & Zainal, 2010) in any type of cancer are related with creating anxiety as well as depression. There are evidences indicating a conditioning of patient with the hospital, hospital bed, the attendant, the doctor, nurses and the like. All this leads to anticipatory nausea and vomiting before chemotherapy; thus deteriorating the quality of life and well-being of cancer patients.

Hospital anxiety can also have a negative impact of leaving the patients untreated. If the prevalent cancer/hospital associated anxiety or depression are not treated there is a very bright chance that the patients may not continue the treatment either due to the fatigue or lack of motivation (Nikbakhsh, Moudi, Abbasian, & Khafri, 2014). At the same time it is not noteworthy that the prevalence of hospital anxiety and depression is quite high (Nikbakhsh, Moudi, Abbasian, & Khafri, 2014). This anxiety can be mild being symptomatic or clinical in nature that may vary in various types of cancer (Nikbakhsh, Moudi, Abbasian, & Khafri, 2014).A correlation of depression, anxiety and QOL with perceived social support was studied amongst the breast cancer patients over a period of 12 months by using HADS, QLQ C-30 version and the multidimensional scale of perceived social support. It was observed that the treatment had a positive effect of significantly reducing the anxiety and depression both at 6 and 12 months in comparison to base line. However the depression did not reduce. The overall QOL and MSPSS (Multidimensional scale of perceived social support) were negatively correlated with anxiety and depression (Guan, Mohamad, See, Harun, Maznah Dahlui, Sulaiman, Zainal, & Taib, 2015). Anxiety and depression are associated with diminished health status and substantially lower health-related quality of life persisting over time (Sherbourne, Wells, Meredith, Jackson, Camp, 1996).

Anxiety and depression are studied as cognitive state of mind of the patients while assessing these in relation to cancer. The cognitive symptoms of depression have been considered to be very important and highly relevant while diagnosing as well as during the monitoring of response the treatment (Rackley & Bostwick, 2012). Such cognitive symptoms include a relatively lower or poor self-esteem, lowered hope, feeling of „loss of control", guilt, sense of loss of purpose in life and being a burden on others.

The above concept and discussion lead to a conclusion that it becomes all the more necessary to make efforts to improve the hope and resilience amongst cancer patients so that they can cope with this ghastly disease.

Hope and cancer

Hope is an affective state that promotes the faith in a positive outcome related to any life events and circumstances in life. The opposite is despair on the other end of continuum. Hope refers to a feeling that what is desired can be achieved or that events will turn out for whatever is the best. Snyder (1994), presented his own definition of hope quoting that "Hope is the sum of the mental *will power* and *way power* that one has for one"s goal". He further continues by deliberating upon the following underlying concepts:

a. ***Goals:*** Goals can be some objects, experiences, or outcomes that one may envisage, visualise or may "desire for or may strongly fix in one"s mind". Snyder explains that the goals involving hope can fall at any point between impossible to a sure thing.

b. ***Willpower:*** Willpower carries a measure impetus in cognitive aspects of hope. It pertains to the perception of the „desired goal" as well as the required mental or emotional energy for achieving it. "How well one can comprehend one"s own goal" is an important determining factor of one"s will power. Within the domain of psychology there are methods to train on how to focus on goal, or how to attain one"s desires and wishes. (Fredrickson, 2008).

c. ***Way power:*** Way power is another important constituent that reflects the cognitive road maps and the mental plans which guide towards hopeful thoughts. Individual"s ability to strategize the path through a goal.

Mental willpower and way power for goals constitute the hope as seen by Snyder. Also both the constituents are different. According to Snyder, Rand, & Sigman

(2002), "an individual with will power thinking may not have way power thoughts to their goals". Hope has also been hypothesized as a construct that is closely related to optimism (Snyder, 2000) with the above mentioned components of

(I) the ability to plan pathways to the desired goals despite obstacles, and,

(II) agency or motivation to use these pathways.

Thus hope is expecting to achieve something desired, while optimism is the confidence about the successful outcome of the events and efforts for future. In case of cancer it pertains to successfulness of "saving life" by treatment. Hope involves pathways and thoughts to a proposed goal. Optimism leads to "Expect the best, but it does not necessarily provide any critical thinking about how we are going to arrive at this improved future" (Fredrickson, 2008).

According to Snyder"s theory the hopeful goal-directed behaviour to succeed is usually determined by an interaction of the followings.

- The degree of "value" of goal or outcome.
- Cognition and process regarding the possible pathways to achieve the goal and the expectation about the effectiveness of the planned pathways to meet the goal.
- The individual concept of one"s personal agency and a trust in being able to follow the paths.

These factors depend on past experiences of individual in the cognitive state of individual about the pathways to goal and about agency regarding the capability of the self as author or casual chain of events. Both these factors are based on developmental lessons. Understanding in this way hope in cancer refers to positive or negative emotions one develops about the successfulness of treatment, one"s cognitions about how to fight against it and a faith in one"s own ability to do the needful for this fight. Obviously more the hope more is the chance of survival.

Diagnosis of cancer brings many and varied emotional response (Gibson, 1999), and hope plays a role here. Hope is an important key factor in influencing the adaptation of the cancer patients with the shocking diagnosis (Chaturvedi, Shenoy, Prasad, Senthilnathan, & Premlata, 1996). "Hope consists of positive thinking towards the future and the desire to effort for life." (Kyngas, Mikkonen, Nousiainen, Rytilahti, Seppanen, &Vaattovaara, 2001).

Resilience and cancer

The American Psychological Association (2010) has defined resilience as "The process of acclimatizing well in the face of trauma, tragedy, adversity, threats or even important sources of threat". Thus it is an individual capacity. Initially resilience was conceived as a trait of personality. However, more recently it has been flexibly described as a „developmental process‟ that is not static (Luthar & Suchman, 2000). Resilience is defined as "the baseline characteristics or traits of an individual which are identified at or during first interaction; enabling individual people to thrive in the face of adversity" (Connor, 2006; Richardson, 2002). The basic demographic variables along with personal resources and abilities like hope and optimism, motivation, individual‟s sense of coherence in life i.e., recognizing the world as meaningful and predictable, already existing social support, and a sense of spirituality along with confidence in the capacity and ability to do something determines one‟s resilience (Herth, 1992; Snyder, Irving, & Anderson, 1991). Others have considered it to be a path/trajectory or process of positive adaptation that protects against psychological distresses that may vary over time (Mancini & Bonanno, 2009).

Some mechanisms of resilience can be identical to the baseline characteristics of individuals that may change over the course of disease and illness. For example, ways of coping in an individual may be considered as the inherent baseline characteristics at the point of screening, and if these change after the diagnosis and during the illness, these may now be considered as a mechanism.

Another school of thought is entirely different. As per this third thought on resilience, it is evidence by relatively positive psychosocial functioning, which usually develop as a result of traumatic stress (Rutter, 2006). Thus it is developed through stress and traumas in life. Personal growth, like post traumatic growth and the reduction/absence of psychological distress are the major outcomes of such resilience.

"It is complex and multidimensional ability to recover from hardship or trauma." (Southwick & Charney, 2012). According to Luthar and Suchman (2000), "resilience is a dynamic process that encompassed positive adaptation in serious adversity." Resilience may differ for different events. For example, a teenager might have successfully avoided the delinquency but may not be able to avoid depression. "Resilience is a broad conceptual umbrella term, covering many concepts related to positive patterns of adaptation in the context of adversity." (Masten & Obradovic, 2006). Multiple factors have been found to contribute to resilience: these include personal, genetic and environmental factors. Personal factors include intellectual functioning, cognitive adaptability, positive self- concept, attachment, emotional regulation, optimism, coping, hopefulness, hardiness, resourcefulness, adaptability and spirituality (Joseph & Linley, 2006). Genetic factors refer to development and changes in brain structure and neurobiological system (Cicchetti & Curtis, 2006). The environmental factors and systematic factors, on the other hand may refer to the learning through difficult life events faced by self or significant others (Luther, Cicchetti & Backer, 2000).

Thus "Psychological resilience is understood as individual ability to cope with stresses and adversities." (American Psychological Association, 2008). Keeping cool in the face of difficulty is what psychologists have called resilience. Resilient people are definitely stronger and more adaptive. They are better than non-resilient in to utilizing their strengths and skills to cope and recover from all kinds of problems and difficulties including natural disaster, job loss, financial problem, medical emergency, divorce or the death of a loved one. That is why resilience has also been conceived as way of coping. Adaptation and coping has a positive result of "bouncing back" to an original, normal functioning or not perceiving negative (Benard, 2004). Resilience thus provides a protection from various physical and mental health conditions including anxiety and depression. Resilience may also provide a cover against lack of sociability, bullying or any other type of previous trauma.

Since cancer is a disease accompanied by anxiety, depression, hopelessness etc., resilience can be an important variable to study in relation to cancer. It has already been discussed that cancer and its treatment has its own stressors, including many associated financial, psychological and physiological changes. Resilience can play a key positive role in adaptation of cancer, accepting it, and in coping with the disease, its treatment and side effects. Therefore, it is utmost necessary to promote the resilience and improve the psychosocial functioning of patients of cancer during and after the treatment as suggested by various studies in chapter 2.

In a study of 68 newly diagnosed head and neck cancer patients, both the baseline characteristics like marital status or optimism and the coping strategies characteristics contribute to growth (Llewellyn, Horney, McGurk, Weinman, Herold, Altman, & Smith, 2013). Similarly among breast cancer patients, factors like satisfaction with the medical experience and optimism were found to be associated with reduced distress during treatment as well as during a follow up till 6 years (Lam,Bonanno, Mancini, Ho, Chan, Hung, & Fielding, 2010; Lam, Shing, Bonanno, Mancini, & Fielding, 2012). Similar findings have been reported for the colorectal cancer patients and recurrent ovarian cancer patients (Hou, Law, Yin, & Fu, 2010; Ponto, Ellington, Mellon, & Beck, 2010).

Interventions do promote resilience and may modify the factors influencing the type of trajectory being faced by the patients. Training on stress management, coping skill, mindfulness, and goal setting can bring a noticeable change. Other mechanism is unique to the medical experience itself, for e.g., positive patient- provider communication.

Resilience has been generally considered as being dynamic and potentially modifiable by the proper interventions by Bradshaw, Richardson, Kumpfer, Carlson, & Stanchfield et al., (2007) and by Burton, Pakenham, & Brown (2010).

Coping and Cancer

Lazarus and Folkman (1984) have defined coping as "constantly changing cognitive and behavioural efforts to manage, reduce or tolerate external and/or internal demands that are appraised as taxing or exceeding the resources of the person." Thinking this way, coping is conveniently deemed as a process that is situation specific; a way of handling everyday situations and events in life. According to Lazarus (1991), "people engage in coping when they feel under stress or want to manage a taxing situation." Lazarus and Folkman have further argued that "coping (a) is process-oriented (rather than trait based), (b) should not be confounded with outcomes of these efforts to manage stress and (c) should not confounded with successful environmental mastery, because it focuses mostly on those attempts to master the environment."

Coping has also been defined by Moos and his associates as "a stabilizing factor that can help individuals maintain psychological adaption during stressful periods. It encompasses cognitive and behavioral efforts to reduce or eliminate stressful conditions and associated emotional distress." (Holahan, Moos, & Shaefer, 1996; Moos & Schaefer, 1984, 1986). Snyder and Dinoff (1999) defined coping as "a response aimed at diminishing the physical, emotional and psychological burden that is linked to stressful life events and daily hassles".

Cancer, no doubt is a frightening and dreadful disease, which is well established and well known to people for the intensely with which it leads to debility, defacement or death. Although most of the men and women learn to cope well during treatment, yet it is merely an adaptation while a significant degree of threat remains. The frequency of people facing psychological and financial distress, sadness, and fearfulness and future related anxieties even after the treatment is significantly high. The fatigue caused by the customary regimen of anticancer drugs causes confusion to worsen the situation; leading to a worry of the cancer returning. In spite of being collectivists, disturbances in family relationships including marital disharmonies after diagnosis of cancer are common. Sexual functioning, actual and perceived, are particularly highly vulnerable. Sexual functioning has been often found to be affected negatively by treatments (Brownson, Alavanja, & Hock, 1993).

Vocational disruption is frequent, particularly amongst the patients with chronic discomposure, anxiety and worry from cancer or its treatments. In many organisations the patients may face some discrimination by colleagues or authorities. Alternations in physical appearance may cause disrupted social and recreational activity. Anxieties may erupt even after a successful treatment. All this has necessitated the psychoeducation of the patients at the time of diagnosis and after recovery. Training on more effective coping and life skills can improve the quality of life of cancer patients. Health psychologists are now focusing attention on strengthening the patients and the care takers so that they can cope and adapt with such plethora of adversarial effects of cancer treatment.

Research indicates that some specific ways of coping strategies might be more helpful in effective handling of the cancer related persistent worries. In a study of 603 cancer patients, Dunkel-Schetter, Feinstein, Taylor, & Falke (1992), identified five patterns of effective coping. These are: distancing, focusing on positive, seeking or using social support, cognitive and behavioural escape-avoidances. Using social support, focus on positive, and distancing were found to be positive ways of coping which dimmed the emotional distress from cancer. On the other hand, cognitive and behavioral escape-avoidance were found to heighten the emotional distress (Stanton & Snyder, 1993).

The belief in having a „sense of control" over the spread and reoccurrence of disease is an important predictor of the associated distress (Taylor, Lichtman, & Wood, 1984). In a study with 78 breast cancer patients, the women with a higher sense of cognitive controls were reported to be better on adjustment and they experienced lesser anxiety, fear, depression and anger (Taylor, Lichtman, & Wood, 1984)

Managing cancer and even survival is determined by the coping style adopted by patients of (Greer, 1991; Pettingalel, Morris, Greer, & Haybittle, 1985). Psychoeducation, counseling and psychotherapy including existential, cognitive and behaviour therapies, along with systematic desensitization, pain control techniques, relaxation independently or with biofeedback and guided imagery, yoga and meditation, music and art therapy, self-help group support have proved to be good adjuncts or complementary therapies in the management of cancer. (Charalambous, Giannakopoulou, Bozas, Marcou, Kitsios, & Paikousis, 2016; Demiralp, Oflaz, & Komurcu, 2010; Lerman, Rimer, Blumber, Cristinzio, Engstrom, MacElwee, & Seay, 1990; Pathak, Mahal, Kohli & Nibran, 2013; Molassiotis, 2000; Tsitsi, Charalambous, Papastavrou, & Raftopoulo, 2017; Yoo, Ahn, Kim, Kim, & Han, 2005).

Above discussion has evinced that it is not easy to maintain a good or positive mental health for a patient of cancer as they face many adverse changes and might require new ways of coping to manage the disease. This has necessitated the psychological intervention to reduce the multiple kinds of anxiety, depression, side effects of medicines etc. and to improve the quality of life and other well-being of cancer patients. Unfortunately, India is yet lagging behind in accepting the psychology and psychological intervention for promoting mental health. However, spiritual counseling is very popular in India. Therefore, it seems relevant to Progressive muscle relaxation which is seemingly close to meditation in the view of public perception.

Progressive muscle relaxation and cancer

Progressive muscle relaxation (**PMR**) can be a good ways of coping in which individual learns to monitor and control the tension in different sets of muscle. The technique came as a boon given by Jacobson in the early 1920s (Jacobson, 1938) after working for long years till before he died infect.

It is a method of sequentially tensing and relaxing of major skeletal muscles in a given specified order that can also be varied. This simple exercise eases both the mind and the body by tensing and relaxing various muscle groups in a progressive manner to reach over the full body. The individual tenses each muscle group briskly for about 5 seconds, without straining, before releasing the self-created tension. Most pertinent is individuals"focus upon taking a serious note of the differences between the state of tensing and relaxing the muscle.

It cannot be a natural human response to remain relaxed when there is a threat from any internal or external stimulant, yet in case of loss of control, the best response of the body would be „no negative response" (Craske & Barlow, 2006). This „no negative response" to stress or threat can be learnt through JPMR. In fact amongst many type of relaxation techniques, JPMR has always persisted as the most popular technique with modern therapists (Craske & Barlow, 2006).

The initial version of Jacobson was too long and was later modified by himself after trying various combinations of muscles (Jacobson, 1938). Now it usually employs 8 sets of muscles. Bio feedback is a modification where in the external devices are used to display the extent of relaxation and then to learn practice to relax without any such support.

The procedure of PMR is scientific and is based on psychobiological principals. It is over all proven that neuromuscular hypertension is the basic cause of a variety of unwanted emotional states leading to many psychosomatic maladies; thus causing the muscle tensions in body that results from anxiety- provoking events and thoughts (Isa, Moy, Razack, Zainuddin, & Zainal, 2013). Though cognitive and physiological pathways underlying the negative emotion are quite intricate, and the precise mechanism of action may not be completely certain, yet muscular relaxation techniques have been undoubtedly effective in lowering down the muscle tension in the body (Conrad & Roth, 2007) and bringing an effective relaxation on state of mind in the practicing individuals. The procedure, if followed successfully, alters the sympathetic nervous system activity. This, in turn, decreases in blood pressure, heart/pulse rate and also the musculoskeletal tone (Chaudhuri, Ray, Saldanha, & Bandopadhyay, 2014). Neuroendocrine functions are also transformed by this method upon achieving a state of relaxation. This seems to be an all evasive kind of method as it relieves anxiety (Curran, 2010), reduces stress (Agee, Danoff-Burg, and Grant. 2009), prevents epileptic seizures (Jain, Batra, Sharma, & Dahiya, 2011), improves sleep and much more.

It has been recommended that deep somatic restfulness reduces anxiety and physical arousal (Payne & Donaghy, 2010). Such relaxation amongst the cancer patients may directly reduce and prevent the anxiety and muscular activity, which usually precedes retching and nausea. By learning of relaxation people perceive a better sense of control on the side effects, thus lowering the anxiety (Payne & Donaghy, 2010).

Some of the researchers have argued that PMR may assist as a distraction for patients undergoing chemotherapy, (Arakawa, 1997), while others argue that distraction is only part of the effectiveness of such interventions (Kwekkeboom, Wanta, & Bompus, 2008). Whatever be the mechanics of action by PMR, the above discussion establishes a confidence of every chance of improvement in the cancer associated symptoms, fatigue and anxiety.

With this background of understanding the meaning and implications of cancer in positive mental health of patients, next chapter reviews the studies pertaining to cancer and mental health.

CHAPTER II

HISTORICAL REVIEW

In the last chapter all theoretical concepts have been described and discussed in details. The present chapter is a review of the past studies on the variables taken in the present piece of research in relation to cancer. Studies have been presented in a chronological manner. The following section deals with the review of quality of life, subjective well-being, hope, resilience, ways of coping, fatigue, hospital anxiety & depression and progressive muscle relaxation as related with cancer of any type. Very old studies have not been included in the chapter due to the paucity of space and lesser relevance in sense of now being confirmatory. The review presents a picture of „cancers as one disease" more than the specific cancers as taken up in the present study. In fact most of the studies have taken into account either single diagnosis of patients as a sample of investigation in a study or all cancers in a group than the investigating specific types of cancer. Breast cancer has been focused quite largely followed by relatively less studies on cervix, prostrate and lung cancers. The review includes such studies also though these were limited in number. After review on each variable, the obtained results have been summarized very briefly at the end of each section.

First of all studies related to quality of life and cancer have been tabulated in Table 2.1

Table 2.1: Showing a review of the studies related quality of life and cancer

Authors and year	Variables	Results
Montazeri, Milory, McEwen, & Gills, (2001).	Cancer survivors and Quality of life (QOL).	Descriptive analyses indicated that perception of symptom and stress play a great role. Those who died within three months perceived that they suffered from significantly worse health problems and Symptom severity. Their perception about their physical functioning, role functioning and overall quality of life was significantly poor than those who survived.
Sprah, & Sostaric, (2004).	Psychosocial problems, coping strategies and cancer patients.	The meta analysis of review did not present any scientific evidence of the effect of coping styles on the initiation of the cancer and its progression and recurrence. However, the psychosocial interventions were shown to have an important role in improvement of quality of life of the cancer patients.
Henoch, Bergman, Gustasson, Gaston-Johansson, & Danielson, (2007).	Quality of life, over time &influence of symptoms, and lung cancer patients.	Amongst lung cancer patients, dyspnea, depression and global quality of life were found to increase overtime. All or all but one follow up measurement

		indicated that performance status as socio demographic anxiety, depression, components of dyspnea, pain as the disease related and the meaningfullness components, coping capacity as a coping measure highly correlated with global quality of life. Multivariate analysis was employed and the global quality of life was taken as the end variable. The analysis revealed depression to be a significant predictor of quality of life. Same results were confirmed in 4 out of 5evaluations. On the other hand coping capacity, anxiety, performance status, pain and social support, though had a significant influence on the quality of life, but this impact was not always consistent and was significant at one or two measures/ evaluations only. Emotional distress and coping capacity as the factors influencing quality of life have been suggested to be the goals for intervention in the palliative care.

Akin, Can, Aydiner, & Durna, (2010).	QOL, the disease-related factors and lung cancer patients.	The quality of Life of lung cancer patients was low in this study. The subscales of health scale and functioning were the lowest on QOL with mean and SD of 20.33 ± 5.59, while those of the family subscales with a value of 27.66 ± 2.77 were the highest. Loss of energy and appetite with additional nausea, coughing, pain were some of the key factors related to the disease that significantly affected the QOL scores. The common psychological symptoms included having difficulty in sleeping, feeling nervous and sad or wretched. Persistent sense of worrying was also a significant concern. The symptom distress and quality of life scores were found to negatively correlate with a value of -0.45 significant at 0.000. The symptom stress was higher in female patients.

Yang, Cheville, Wampfler, Garces, Jatoi, Clark, (2012).	QOL, and lung cancer patients.	In a 7-year longitudinal in primary lung cancer survivors were found to suffer from a substantial symptom burden. QOL was significantly impaired. The researchers suggested implementing the target interventions in order to reduce the symptoms burden amongst lungs cancer survivors.
Torkzahrani, Rastegari, Khodakarami, Akbarzadeh-Baghian, & Alizade, (2013).	QOL, socio-demographic variables, social support & disease related factors and Cervix Cancer (CC) patients,	Cervix cancer patients reported a good QOL, though it was negatively associated with disease related symptoms like reduced hunger, treatment related nausea and vomiting, being short of breath or breathing problems, sleep related issues, and menopausal symptoms. QOL was found to be positively correlated with economic conditions and social functioning amongst cervix cancer patients.

Khalil, Sahli, Afif, Elkacemi, Elmajjaoui, Kebdani,& Benjaafar, (2015).	General & sexual QOL, and cervix cancer survivors (CCS).	In spite of a good global QLQ, CCS expressed issues concerning emotional functioning and less sexual functioning enjoyment. Less satisfaction with their body image was experienced by CCS in comparison to healthy controls.
Pandey, Dhungana, Twi, Byanju, & Khawas, (2015).	Cancer Patients and Quality of life.	The quality of Life amongst cancer patients was found to be relatively better in the present study. Some aspects were rated higher by some patients like physical, cognitive, emotional and role functioning while others were lower on some e.g., social functioning. Many factors were reported to influence the QOL of cancer patients like the cancer cite, its stage and time after diagnosis. The average QOL scores on different scales were 85.54 on global health/QOL, 77.03 on functional, and 16.14 on associated symptom scale out of 100. The most frequent complaint was the loss of appetite (mean = 20.27); indeed amongst almost all the patients. Scores on various QOL scales

		like physical, cognitive, emotional, social, role functioning as well as pain, fatigue or dyspnea, loss of appetite and nausea /vomiting and even the financial problems were found to be significantly correlated with overall QOL of the patients.
Pradhan, Sarkar, & Lakshminarayanan, (2015).	Socio-demographic, disease characteristic, QOL, and cervix cancer patients.	Overall QOL was found to be poor in a greater proportion of patients of cervical cancer. Psychological domain was the found to be worst (71%). Uneducated, widowed, postmenopausal and the survivors with recurrence of disease were found to be at an increased risk of having poor QOL.

Dahiya, Acharya, Bachani, Sharma, Gupta, Haresh, & Rath, (2016).	QOL, chemotherapy, radiotherapy and cervical Cancer patients.	Six months survival of cervical patients was found to be good and the treatment had a significant improvement on global health as the pre score increased from 50.15 to 59.52 after six months and was significant (p= .00007) was 92.53%. Physical, cognitive and emotional functioning had also improved significantly (p<0.05). Fatigue, pain, insomnia and appetite loss but episodes of diarrhea had increased after the treatment. The mean "symptoms score" after treatment being 20.0 was significantly lower than the pretreatment score being 30.0. This difference was highly significant, that is, at the level of 0.00001. Both the sexual functioning and enjoyment had significantly reduced after treatment.
Polanski, Jankowska-Polanska, Rosinczuk, Chabowski, & Szymanska-Chabowska, (2016).	Lung cancer patients and QOL.	Comparison was made with healthy population as well as patients suffering from other malignancies and the quality of life in lung cancer patients was much lower. The severity and the number of symptoms i.e. fatigue,

		loss of appetite, dyspnea, cough, pain and blood in sputum largely affected the quality of life of these patients. Fatigue and respiratory problems were found to reduce the psychological dimensions of quality of life, while sleep problems were found to reduce the cognitive functioning. Decrease in physical dimension related to growing disability and on inability to play the required family and social roles amongst majority were the serious concerns and cancer as amongst such patients.
Vashistha, Singh, Kaur, Prokop, & Kaushik, (2016).	Fatigue, QOL, depression & anxiety, exercise interventions and Prostate Cancer patient.	An intervention of 12-16-weak exercise significantly improved upon the fatigue symptoms (MD 4.83, 95% CI 3.24-6.43; $p<0.00001$). At a follow up after 6 months the effect on fatigue was found to be intact as yet (MD 3.60, 95% CI 2.80-5.12; $p<0.00001$). The QOL of prostate cancer patients in general also improved by the given exercise interventions (MD 3.93, 95% CI 1.37-5.92; $p = 0.003$) and also when measured upon Prostate scale (MD 3.85, 95% CI 1.25-

		6.46; p=0.04). The pooled data, however, did not reveal any significant improvement in the initial levels of anxiety or depression.
Engl, Drescher, Bickeboller, & Gradhorn, (2017).	Fatigue, depression, QOL and prostate cancer patients treated with Androgen, Deprivation Therapy (ADT) and in patients with Lower Urinary Tract Symptoms (LUTS) and prostate cancer Patients.	Both the groups did not differ in terms of fatigue (BFI). Amongst the prostate cancer patients, EORTC-QLQ-C30 role function was found to be highly and significantly impaired. Fatigue score was also higher. Differences on the BDI in regards to self-criticism were observed and the mean scores for LUTS patients were higher. On the other hand, loss of energy and loss of sexual interest were more relevant for prostate cancer patients. But the differences were not significant.

The studies have shown a trend of reducing the QOL of cancer patients on various indicators. The results of EORTC-QLQ-C30 have shown a consistent trend of reduced QOL in total and its various dimensions i.e. functional status, symptom status and global health status. Besides this, other indicators like overall performance, sleep and its quantity, anxiety, pain, coping capacity which are known to be the factors affecting the QOL were also affected negatively by cancer. The socio demographic variables like income, occupation, education and status of being single were also related with the effect of cancer on QOL. Health related QOL was also found to negatively affect.

Hope, social support and presence of care taker were also the variables that played a role in the determining the QOL. Severity, stage and presence of symptoms were amongst such other factors.

The next section of studies is about well-being. The terms Health related quality of life and well-being have been used interchangeably by researchers. Some studies of health related quality of life (HRQOL) have already been presented in the above section. Following section deals with the studies that have used FACT-G as assessment tool that measures physical, functional, emotional and social well-being while Cella, (1993) who developed this tool has called it as the overall score of HRQOL. Studies related to well-being and cancers are tabulated in table 2.2.

Table 2.2: Showing a review of the studies related to well-being and cancer

Authors and year	Variables	Results
Holzner, Kemmler, Cella, De Paoli, Meraner, Kopp, Greil, Fleischhacker, & Sperner-Unterweger, (2004)	HRQOL, and breast cancer survivors & Survivors of Hodgkin"s disease.	Of the total questionnaires distributed, 968 questionnaires were received back; thus comprising a large sample for investigation. 48.3% were the females with a mean age of 49.39 years. The level of education had a significant impact and more educated patients reported higher HRQOL. Poor marital status in terms of either being divorced or being a widow had a significantly negative lower score on such quality of life. Ageing played a significant role and the HRQOL of elderly was found to be poor. Most of the patients were poor on QOL even after bone marrow transplantation when compared with a matched control group (age and sex).

		Interestingly, the social well-being of breast cancer survivors was significantly reduced while amongst the survivors of Hodgkin"s disease functional and social well-beings were significantly higher than the normal healthy controls. The researchers have recommended that the Socio-demographic variables are important indicators of HRQOL.
Humpel, & Iverson, (2007).	Well-being and breast & prostate cancer patients.	Physical activity amongst both types of cancer patients was found to be decreased significantly decreased from pre to post diagnosis. Contrarily 20.9% of the patients recounted their activity levels to have improved after the diagnosis. More than 30% patients in the total sample reported them to be depressed. With a slight difference in frequencies the improvement was significant amongst breast cancer participants on all the dimensions of physical well-being, emotional well-being and functional well-being. When tested upon $\chi 2$ (6.83, $p < .04$), it was found that those not involved in physical activity were more depressed than who involved them in physical activity. Thus physical activity amongst oncology patients can

		improve upon their well-being.
Ardebil, Bouzari, Shenas , Zeinalzadeh, & Barat, (2011).	Depression, health related quality of life (HRQOL), and women with breast cancer.	More than half of patients reported depression and all domains of HRQOL were found to be negatively affected by depression. Significant differences were found between depression and treatment type. More participants in the chemotherapy group, suffered from depression than in the radiotherapy group. Statistically significant effects of depression were reported in overall HRQOL. Participants with depression were more likely to have poorer overall HRQOL, except social and family well-being. The authors suggested and recommended the necessity of implementing the health strategies in breast cancer patients.
Benbrahim, Fakir, Mrabti, Nejjari, Benider, Errihani, Mesbani, & Mellas, (2016).	Health Related Quality of Life, and Lung Cancer patients.	Health related quality of Life was found to be impaired in comparison to the normal control subjects. However social functioning was an exception with higher mean score (77.7 vs. 71.3). QLQ-LC13, measured lung cancer associated symptoms. The symptoms were found to be more severe particularly for dyspnea, coughing and chest pain. Poorer health related quality was found amongst the patients with lower performance status and

		advanced stage disease.
Ahmed, Nahla, Nivine, Amal, & Ibrahim, (2016).	Health related quality of life and breast cancer patients.	The Functional domain was found to be least affected, whereas the physical domain were found to be most seriously affected in breast cancer patients. Significant socio-demographic variables affecting the quality of life included the age of patient, level of education, number of children and total family income. Presence of care giver proved to be a key factor; while affecting the different dimensions of HRQOL differently. The age of patient at the time of diagnosiswas also a disease-related factors affecting HRQOL along with the post-operative chemotherapy, an inability to stick to the treatment regimen in terms of medication and the affection in the side of the predominant hand.
Fleming, Ramirez, Soliman, Schemeler, Chisholm, Nick, Westin, & Frumovitz, (2016).	Functional Assessment of Cancer Therapy-Cervix (FACT-Cx), QOL, symptom assessment, Female Sexual	The Functional assessment on arousal, lubrication, orgasm, pain, satisfaction and total score were found to be significantly poor when assessed at 6 weeks. However, such changes were found to be temporary and these returned to baseline levels by six months. The FACT-Cx assessment also showed a significant worsening of

	Functioning Index, Satisfaction with Decision and cervical cancer patients.	the physical well- being along with functioning and role physical and functional well-being, SF-12 bodily pain, role emotional and social functioning at the post assessment of six weeks, which again resumed the baseline levels at an assessment after half a year. However, the longitudinal study indicated the significant worsening of symptoms on emotional well-being on multiple measures taken till four years. There was no difference in satisfaction with decision.
Harju, Rantanen, Kaunonen, Helminen, Isotalo, & Astedt-kurki, (2018).	Health-related quality of life and prostate cancer patients.	The HRQOL of the prostate cancer patients along with their spouses was found to be better on all dimensions, i.e., physical, functional and emotional when compared with the general population. Patients age, manifestation of disease, and the method of treatment were the key factors found to be associated with various dimensions of HRQOL. At the same time the age, education (both basic and vocational) and the status of disease of the spouse were also found to play a significant role in HRQOL of these patients.

Overall health related QOL and well- being has been reported to consistently reduce with cancer. All types of well -being, that is, emotional, functional and physical or symptoms related well- being were negatively affected. Some studies have shown a strong role of socio demographic variables in determining the well -being/ HRQOL.

Fatigue is another important variable that is well established to accompany the cancer by tooth and nail. It is a major symptom that affects both the QOL and well-being in routine. Biologically the body demands some rest and at the same time fatigue is psychologically debilitating. This might lead to double negative effect in the cancer patients; in a sense by creating additional burden of fatigue in cancer along with its own burden. The next table 2.3 shows the review of studies related to fatigue and cancer.

Table 2.3: Showing a review of the studies related to fatigue and cancer

Authors and year	Variables	Results
Stone, Richards, Ahem, & Hardy, (2000).	Fatigue, QOL and cancer patients.	Assessed the existence of fatigue, its severity as well as its correlation among the patient of cancer in comparison to control group. They found that, the degree of fatigue varied amongst various type of cancer. Being 78% it was much higher in the lung cancer patient in comparison to 15% and 16% in the patient cancer and prostate cancer respectively.
Jereczek-Fossa, Marsiglia, & Orecchia, (2002).	Fatigue and prostate & breast cancer patients.	Radiotherapy in itself is a process that can induce fatigue. It was observed that the physiological mechanism were responsible for such fatigue in early breast cancer and prostate cancer patients. Neuromuscular efficiency was found to reduce. It was also found that physical exercise and relaxation

		helped the patients in getting rid of the accompanying fatigue in cancer.
Visovsky, & Schneider, (2003).	Fatigue and lung cancer women patients.	It was found in this study that, fatigue was at the top to create distress in the lung cancer women patients. Being most frequent it was also twice as high pain in these patients. They also concluded that it reduced the quality of life as well as the physical, functional, symptoms. Therefore symptoms management required.
Goedendorp, Gielissen, Verhagen, Peters, & Bleijenberg, (2008).	Fatigue, pain physical activity and prostate, breast & gastrointestinal cancer patients.	An effort was to make to understand that which factors are contributing to fatigue by taking various type of cancer before the diagnosis. 14.3% of prostate cancer, 20.3% of breast cancer, 28.1% of gastro intestine cancer patients reported severe level of fatigue. The current factor included impairment in sleep and rest, depressive mood and level of physical activity. The factors affecting before the diagnosis was the fatigue experienced during last one year before the diagnosis.
Mendoza, Laudico, Wang, Guo, Matsuda, Yosuico, Fragante, & Charles, (2010).	Fatigue and cancer patients.	The degree of fatigue was assessed in the cancer patients. Only 17% patients were found to have severe level of fatigue, 34% suffered from moderate level of fatigue, 49% of patients regarded to have mild fatigue.

Borneman, Piper, Koczywas, Munevar, Sun, Uman, & Ferrell, (2012).	Fatigue and prostate cancer patients.	This was a qualitative study to understand cancer related fatigue (CRF). CRF was found to have a highly impact upon the daily activity of cancer patients. It reduced all type of well-being including physical, psychological and spiritual. This not only limited the ability of patient to function and socialize but also changed the meaning of suffering and cancer related experiences.
Langston, Armes, Levy, Tidey, & Ream, (2013).	Fatigue and prostate cancer patients.	The distressing symptom of the fatigue in the patients of prostate cancer was studied by reviewing 19 pieces of research. 17 of these were cross-sectional whereas 2 were longitudinal studies. It was found that prevalence of fatigue was very high that is 74%. When radiotherapy was combined with hormone therapy. The prevalence of fatigue was found to be higher that is 39%.
Sekse, Huffthammer, & Vika, (2015).	Fatigue and Gynecological cancer patients.	Gynecological cancer was studied to understand the fatigue in women. 53% of the women reported cancer related fatigue which was higher in cervix cancer patient followed by the patient"s of ovarian cancer. Age was found to have no impact.
Nautiyal, Lal, Verma, Yadav, Singh, & Kumar, (2015).	Fatigue, QOL and Head & Neck cancer patients.	Assessed the level of fatigue in the head and neck cancer which was found to be significantly higher than the control group. However the treatment given by radiotherapy reduced the fatigue by three

		month. By 12 month they had recovered from the fatigue.
Carnio, Di Stefano, & Novello, (2016).	Fatigue and lung cancer patients.	Lung cancer patient were studied to understand the fatigue related to cancer. It was concluded that fatigue in the cancer patients belongs to a cluster of symptoms including depression, insomnia and pain. Irrespective of the stage of lung cancer physical exercise was suggested to be the best way to cope.
Steen, Dahl, Hess, & Kiserud, (2017).	Fatigue and cervix cancer patients.	A longitudinal study was conducted on fatigue in long term survivor of cervix cancer. 23% of the patients reported fatigue after diagnosis. These patients also reported more associated symptom like heart disease or blood pressure etc.

To summarize, the fatigue has been reported to vary with type of cancer. Lung cancer and cervix cancer seem to be more fatigued than other types. Radiotherapy was found to reduce the neuromuscular efficiency and QOL of these patients. The perception of the disease as well as behavioral and emotional factors like mood, depression and level of activity were found to be associated with fatigue in cancer patients. Well-being and hope were also found to be affected by fatigue. In fact along with physical well-being emotional, spiritual well-being was also affected. Age had no effect on the level of hope. Most of the studies have recommended that level of activity should be enhanced.

It has been discussed in the above section that cancer brings with it anxiety and depression which reduce the QOL and well-being of the patients. Hospital anxiety is slightly different from the routine or disease related anxiety. It pertains to the conditioning with the negative stimuli in the hospital particularly with reference to chemo and radiotherapy. Following section deals with the studies pertaining to **Hospital anxiety and depression.** Studies related to hospital anxiety & depression and cancer have been tabulated in table 2.4.

Table 2.4: Showing a review of the studies related to hospital anxiety & depression and cancer

Authors and year	Variables	Results
Aass, Fossa, Dahl, & Aloe, (1997).	Anxiety, depression and cancer patients.	HADS and EORTC QOL C-33 were used to assess the prevalence anxiety and depression amongst 716 patients of cancer. The outdoor patients were as less as twice on the risk on psychiatric distress then the hospitalized patients. The males and the elderly patients were also lesser were at a higher risk of anxiety than females than younger patients. However, depression was not associated with age or gender. Anxiety and depression were also found to lead to impaired abilities to continue with early life activity and social life as these were found to improve the physical functioning, fatigue and pain. Fatigue was found to predict depression. Whereas anxiety was predictive by female gender and impaired physical activity as well as social role.

Groenvold, Fayers, Spranger, Bjorner, Klee, Aaronson, Bech, & Mouridsen, (1999).	Anxiety, depression and breast cancer patients.	538 newly diagnosed breast cancer patients who were at a lower risk of recurrence were compared to 872 normal women by using HADS. The occurrence of anxiety and depression did not differ significantly in the two groups. However, it is not very appropriate to use HADS.
Malekian, Alizadeh, & Ahmadzadeh (2007).	Anxiety, depressionand cancer patients.	The levels of anxiety and depression were found to be moderate and high respectively being 18.5% and 32.9%. Anxiety had higher prevalence among cancer patients. Age and gender did not show any correlation with depression. Prevalence of depression and anxiety were not found to be correlated with type of malignancy, treatment duration and the treatment method used for these patients.
Schwarz, Krauss, Hockel, Meyer, Zenger, & Hinz, (2008).	Anxiety, depression and cancer patients.	The patients of breast and gynecological cancer were studied to assess the causes of anxiety and depression over time and to find out the factors that determine the changes in the level of both. Repeated measures on HADS were taken in the beginning after 6 month, after 12 months and the end of the treatment in the hospital. The anxiety and depression were at the peak in the beginning in treatment or the stay in the hospital. After one year the score of depression came down to equal the normal population. The

		treatment, time after diagnosis and education were found to be accountable for this decline. However, the score on anxiety did not change and remain elevated longer time and lower education level were considered to be the high risk factors found in anxiety and depression.
Dogar, Azeem, Kiran, Hussain, Mehmood, & Hina, (2009).	Depression, anxiety and cancer patients.	60 diagnosed cancer patients were assessed on Hospital anxiety and depression scale (HADS) and DSM-IV criterion of assessment of anxiety and depression. Anxiety, depression or both were found to be high in 52% of cancer patients (10 male + 21 female =31). 14 patients exhibited anxiety (6 male + 8 female), 6 patients have shown depression (2 male + 4 female). Whereas 11 patients had both depression and anxiety (2 male +9 female). In this way females had shown a higher prevalence of anxiety, depression or both. As the prevalence up to 70% in females against 33% in the male cancer patients.
Saniah, & Zainal, (2010).	Coping strategies, depression, anxiety and breast cancer patients.	Breast cancer patients undergoing chemotherapy were given HADS and the brief cope scale (149 patients). The prevalence of anxiety (24.1%) was more than the depression (19.1%). The patients with higher anxiety adopted denial, venting and behavioral disengagement

		more than those who were low on anxiety. On the other hand the depressive patients used behavioral disengagement and self-blame, being significantly higher than those low on depression.
Farooqi, & Chaudhry, (2012).	Depression, anxiety and breast & uterus cancer patients.	Breast cancer and uterus cancer patients were taken to asses them on HADS. The patients of uterus cancer were found to be significantly higher on depression and anxiety than the breast cancer patients. These were not correlate significantly with age, education and during of cancer. It is recommended that psychological intervention should be included in the treatment and the rehabilitation in the cancer patient.
Nikbakhsh, Moudi, Abbasian, & Khafri, (2014).	Anxiety, depression and cancer patients.	HADS was used to assess the level of anxiety and depression amongst recently diagnosed patients of different type of cancer. 29.3% patients were found to suffer from mild anxiety and 16.7% had symptomatic anxiety. The depression was relatively high 26.7% suffered from mild depression and 21.3% suffered from symptomatic depression. Older patients had significantly higher prevalence of anxiety and depression. Besides age and type of cancer was also an important factor the higher prevalence of anxiety and depression was found in breast and

		stomach cancer patients then the other type of cancer.
Srivastava, Ansari, Kumar, Shah, Meena, Sevach, & Singh, (2014).	Socio-economic factors, anxiety, depression, psychological distress and breast cancer patients.	The study was conducted on 200 patients diagnosed for having breast cancer. The hospital anxiety and depression scale (HADS) was given twice i.e. immediately, when diagnosed and 12 months after the completion of the treatment. Anxiety (37%) and depression (28%) were highly prevalent. Anxiety was found to be strongly associated with age, level of education, monthly income and financial support. Higher the age, lower the incomes, level of education and financial support high was the anxiety. Similarly low income, being single and less financial support was associated with higher depression after 12 month both the anxiety and depression has reduced.
Guan, Mohamad, Hoong, Harun, Dahlui, Hatim, Zuraida, & Taib, (2015).	Depression, anxiety, quality of Life (QOL), Perceived Social Support and breast cancer women.	A correlation of depression, anxiety and QOL with perceived social support was studied amongst the breast cancer patients over a period of 12 months by using HADS, QLQ C-30 version and the multidimensional scale of perceived social support. It was observed that the treatment had a positive effect of significantly reducing the anxiety and depression both at 6 and 12 months in comparison to base line. However the

		depression did not reduce. The overall QOL and MSPSS (Multidimensional scale of perceived social support) were negatively correlated with anxiety and depression.
Hassan, Shah, Ghazi, Mohd Mujar, Samsuri, & Baharom, (2015).	Anxiety, depression and breast cancer patients.	The analysis of 205 breast cancer patients indicated the prevalence of anxiety to be 31.7% and depression to be 22%. Age, income and number of visit were significantly associated with anxiety, showing that the patients who were younger and had lower monthly income were as likely as twice to be associated with anxiety. Depression was found to be associated with marital status, financial support, family support in turning of a caring person and the felt burden. Depression was likely to be 3-4 times more associated with lower level of income and being single.
Diana, Leong, & Gingin, (2016).	Anxiety, depression, lymphoma survivors and quality of life.	156 lymphoma survivors were assessed on HADS and EORTC QLQ C-30. 18% of the patients suffered from anxiety symptoms whereas 10% had shown the symptom of depression. Older age and lower education were associated with higher level of depression whereas anxiety was associated with lower quality of life, lower emotional and cognitive functioning and higher level of fatigue.

		The depressive patients were also found to be lower as physical functioning and also suffered from insomnia.
Kumar, Singh, Rae, Singh, & Singh, (2016).	Anxiety, depression and cancer patients.	The researchers feel that there is a need to develop an evidence based practice to introduce interventions as untreated anxiety and depression can lead to significant morbidity. The results of their study pictured the prevalence of anxiety and depression among all types of cancer patients. Accordingly, a „continuous screening for anxiety and depression" was recommended by them as a necessary ingredient for good cancer care.
Paul, Musa, & Chungu, (2016).	Depression, quality of life and Cervical cancer patients.	102 cervix cancer patients undergoing the treatment were assessed to identify the risk factor for depression and its effect upon quality of life. The prevalence of depression was found to be quite high. 78% of the patients showed moderate, 18% showed mild and 4% showed severe depression assessed on Back"s Depression Inventory. It suggested that early diagnosis, treatment, care and support would benefit the quality of life of these patients.

The hospital anxiety and depression were found to be high in all type of cancer patients studied in the past. However, the trend of reducing this anxiety and depression seems to be consistent by the end of treatment and it starts reducing after the treatment begins. Some studies show a negative effect of old age whereas other do not. Other socio demographic variable like family support, level of incomes etc. were also found to be amongst the factor affecting the level of hospital anxiety and depression. Anxiety and depression have been reported to have a negative effect on mental health variable like QOL, well-being and sleep etc. on many studies it has been recommended to integrate the intervention to reduce the anxiety and depression as treatment of cancer patients.

The next section of review is related to hope and cancer. **Hope** is an essential ingredient of life that first develops a trust that one can recover from a ghastly disease of cancer and then provides a goal to work upon how to cover. The studies related to hope and cancers are tabulated in table 2.5.

Table 2.5: Showing a review of the studies related to hope and cancer

Authors and year	Variables	Results
Berendes, Keefe, Somers, Kothadia, Porter, & Cheavens, (2010).	Hope, multiple indices of adjustment and lung cancer.	The major physical symptoms considered in the study were fatigue, pain and cough while psychological symptoms included distress, i.e. depression. After taking the key demographic variables and other medical variables into account (e.g., age and stage of cancer etc.) hope was found to be inversely related to these symptoms indicating that more the symptoms lower the hope.
Denewer, Farouk, Mostafa, & Elshamy, (2011).	Hope, social support and breast cancer.	301 women were newly diagnosed of breast cancer were contacted for filling up the special questioner to study hope and social support amongst these

		patients. Structured interview were also taken. 103 patients (34%) women had a low degree of hope, 109 patients (36.2%) had a moderate degree of hope and only 89 patients (29.6%) had a relatively higher degree of hope. Similarly social support was also reported to be relatively low. 81 patients (26.9%) had high, 101 patients (33.6%) had moderate and 119 patients (39.5%) had a low degree of social support. The study did not indicate any significant difference in social support and hope in relation to socio demographic variable age (21-88), educational status, marital status and residence.
Rajandram, Samuel, Samman, Chan, McGrath, & Zwahlen, (2011).	Hope, optimism, anxiety, depression and cancer patients.	Hope, in the present study was negatively and significantly correlated with depression amongst cancer patients as well as anxiety. Pattern of correlation of optimism with the latter adjustment outcomes was very similar. Regression analyses was also applied, which identified hope and optimism as significant predictors of depression. Both the variables had almost equal association with depression. Hope and optimism together significantly predicted anxiety, whereas when tested alone, neither hope nor optimism proved to be

		significant predictor of anxiety.
Oztunc, Yesil, Paydas, & Erdogan, (2013).	Hopelessness, social support and breast cancer patients.	The study targeted upon understanding and identifying social support and hopelessness amongst the breast cancer patients undergoing treatment in various hospitals. The hopelessness scales were found to be low whereas patient"s social support scores were found to be high. Also a linear but reverse relationship between social support and hopelessness was observed. Hopelessness was found to be significantly related with level of education (of the spouse), income, occupation and the number of children.
Wakiuchi, Marchi, Norvila, Marcon, & Sales, (2015).	Hope and cancer patients.	The initially low levels of hope were found to enhance towards the end of the treatment, but this increase was not significant. Level of education, presence of metastases, treatment mode/s and the absence or reduction of moderate to strong pain were found to be the major factors that influenced hope.
Karampour, Fereidooni-Moghadam, Zarea, & Masoudi, (2017).	Hope and cancer patients.	Hope was investigated in 118 breast cancer patients more of the patients found to have a moderate level of hope in the patient taken from south west of Iran. No significant relationship with various socio demographic variables was observed.

Li, Lin, Liang, Hu, Chen, Lan, Liang, Zeng, Wang, & Fu, (2017).	Hope, Psychological health status, psychological distress, functional distress and cervical cancer patients undergoing radiotherapy.	Most of the patients exhibited either moderate or high levels of hope while undergoing radiotherapy. Hope levels amongst oncology patients undertaken in this study were negatively correlated with the Psychological distress index of these patients. QOL of cervix cancer patients varied from moderate to high level and correlated positively with optimism, appeasement, and self-reliance. On the other hand, QOL was negatively correlated with emotional expression and belief of predestination.

To summarize, the past studies related to hope have established that hope was consistently found to reduce amongst the cancer patients. When the initial levels were measured majority of the studies showed that hope was low, though moderate level of hope were also reported in some studies. The hope was not found to be correlated with socio demographic variables in many studies while other studies found contradicting findings. In some studies it was also found to improve after the successful treatment. These and other studies have shown that breast cancer has been studied by most of the researchers and many studies have taken all types of cancer together. It is concluded that hope related interventions are important as the hope and optimism are the variables that have a direct impact upon the mental health variables.

Resilience is another important factor that has as important role in maintaining the positive health as the hope. Resilience acts like a cover against the wear and tear of one"s mental health even in daily life. The more is the resilience better is the adjustment with negative life events. Cancer is also a negative event and resilience is expected to play a highly important role. Following is a review of the earlier work pertaining to resilience and cancer.

Table 2.6: Showing a review of the studies related to resilience and cancer

Authors and year	Variables	Results
Ferreira Filho, Junior, Da Silva, De Souza, Tavares, Cavalcante, & Wunder, (2010).	Resilience and breast cancer patients.	In the group of patients ≥ 50 years age, chemotherapy was more frequently used with palliative purpose (14/16) in comparison to the younger patients (6/13), (P = 0.041). The mean total resilience score was 136 for patients with ≥ 50 years and 143 for patients < 50 years (P = 0.13). No statistical differences in mean resilience were detected between patients receiving palliative or curative chemotherapy (P = 0.2).
Ha, Jung, & Choi, (2014).	Resilience, QOL and breast cancer patients.	Resilience was found to be positively correlated with quality of life of the subjects. Religion and hobby also showed statistically significant difference indication a positive role in resilience. On the other hand Resilience and Post Traumatic Stress Disorder was found to be negatively correlated with QLQ Post Traumatic Stress Disorder and quality of life were negatively correlated. Resilience and PTSD were the variables which explained 44.9% of the variance. Thus resilience plays a positive role in the life of cancer patients.

Kim, Kim, & Lee, (2015).	Resilience and breast cancer patients.	Resilience was significantly but negatively correlated to depression amongst breast cancer patients. However, hope and family support, both had a significantly positive correlation with resilience. Further it is notable that in this study, anxiety was not correlated to resilience. Regression analysis was employed. Hope and religion were the personal factors influencing resilience. Disease related factors included surgery; side and the time elapsed, and lymph node metastasis. All these factors together explained for 34.1% of the variation.
Markovitz, Schrooten, Amtz, & Peter, (2015).	Resilience, emotional response and breast cancer patients.	Cancer patients were reported to have higher levels of anxiety, depression, and negative affect simultaneously having lower levels of positive affect and present happiness when compared to control group of healthy women. Resilience in the two groups did not differ significantly. Higher levels of resilience were related with a relatively superior emotional adjustment both in women with and without breast cancer. However, such an association was much stronger within the cancer patients. Actually the patients scoring high on

		resilience seemed to experience similar levels of anxiety, depression, and the present level of happiness as the healthy women.
Ristevska-Dimitrovska, Filov, Rajchanovska, Stefanovski, & Dejanova, (2015).	Quality of life, Resilience and breast cancer patients.	(i) Correlation of resilience was found to be positive with QLQ and negative with symptom severity. (ii) Body image and future prospective were found to worsen with lower resilience. It was concluded that resilience leads to better quality of life amongst breast cancer patients.
Ristevska-Dimitrovska, Stefanovski, Smichoska, Raleva, & Dejanova, (2015).	Resilience, Depression and breast cancer patients.	The breast cancer patients with lower levels of depression have had higher levels of resilience. It was concluded that the psychological resilience may be contributing independently to lower levels of depression amongst these patients. The level of psychological resilience could be a protective factor for psychological distress and depression
Vartak, (2015).	Hope, social support, resilience and cancer patients.	Results indicate that both hope and social support have a positive and statistically significant impact on the resilience of cancer patients ($p < 0.05$ for hope and social support individually). These findings raised the possibility that intervention at an early stage can increase the resilience and improve the

		mental health of cancer patients.
Giacomo, Cannita, Ranieri, Cocciolone, & Ficorella, (2016).	Psychological resilience, psychological distress and young women breast cancer patients.	The findings showed that young patients seem to be emotionally more resilient i.e., being able to transform the negative emotional experiencing in personal growth. The younger patients can be considered to support with specific treatment for improving their well-being and QOL after overcoming their physical weakness. The two groups study of breast cancer and the normal control group indicated that depression was higher amongst the patients. The anger experiences, its expression and control along with the expression anxiety highlighted resilient performance.
Matzka, Mayer, Köck, Hódi, Moses-Passini, Dubey, Jahn, Schneeweiss, & Eicher, (2016).	Psychological distress, physical activity, resilience and cancer patients.	Cancer patients who are high on resilience, particularly the older patients, were found to experience less psychological distress. Such patients were also observed to be physically more active.
Somasundaram, & Devamani, (2016).	Resilience, social support, & hopelessness and cancer patients treated with	Resilience amongst cancer patients was found to be significantly associated with lower hopelessness and higher perceived social support. In other words if hope is generated and social support is provided,

	curative & palliative care.	the resilience amongst cancer patients can be increased.
Alias & Ravindranadan, (2017).	Job status, resilience and breast cancer patients.	The present study reveals that resilience is comparative. The working patients of cancer were compared with non-working patients with cancer on resilience. One way ANOVA and t test indicated that resilience amongst working patients of breast cancer was significantly higher than non-working breast cancer patients.

Most of the studies have shown that resilience was positively correlated in the QOL of cancer patients. Depression was found to be significantly correlated with resilience. Anxiety was negatively correlated in most of the studies whereas sometimes it was found to have no correlation with resilience. Higher levels of resilience have been considered to be protective factors against depression and psychological distress amongst cancer patients. To mention some other variables resilience was found to be positively correlated with religion, hope, perceived social support and hobbies. Younger and working patients of cancer were reported to be higher on resilience amongst cancer patients in the above studies.

Those high on resilience are expected to cope better with negative life events like cancer, **Coping ways**, styles and strategies have been established as important means towards well- being and happiness in daily life. Ways of coping can be multiple within an individual and have been established to play an important role in management of diseases. Problem focused and emotional focused are two major ways of coping with different styles contained in these two major categories which have been reviewed below for their role in cancer. Table 2.7 shows the studies related to ways of coping and cancer.

Table 2.7: Showing a review of the studies related to ways of coping and cancer

Authors and year	Variables	Results
Reynolds, Hurley, Torres, Jackson, Boyd, & Chen, (2000).	Coping strategies and breast cancer survivors among White & Black women.	The study observed that there is an important role of the coping strategy adopted by the breast cancer survivor. When assessed upon a modified version of Lazarus and Folkman survival was found to be significantly better by the use of emotion focused coping; expression of emotion was positively associated. The subjects with high levels of both the emotional expression and perceived emotional support experienced better survival than those who were low on both.
Kim, Yeom, Seo, Kim, & Yoo, (2003).	Coping Strategies and cancer patients.	62.6% participant in the study suffering from variety of cancer were male and 91.4 % were married. The results indicated that the women oncology patients and the patients in third stage of disease were higher on stress and poorer in coping in the diseases up to then the other groups. Stress was found to correlate negatively with both types of coping i.e. problem or emotion focused coping. The study also indicated that the emotion focused coping was used more by the cancer

		patients than the problem focused coping.
Sehlen, Song, Fahmuller, Herschbach, Lenk, Hollenhorst, Schymura, Aydemir, & Duhmke, (2003).	Coping strategies, psychosocial adaptation and breast cancer patients.	Patients suffering from various types of cancer in the beginning of radiotherapy found to practice a reduced active problem oriented coping and the depressive coping whereas active problem oriented coping and destruction are vital in coping with cancer. Breast cancer patients suffered the most from this. This was found to increase the psycho social distress and lower the QOL. Marital status was also found to have significant influence on spirituality and the active problem oriented coping strategy.
Ransom, Jacobsen, Schmidt, & Andrykowski, (2005).	Ways of coping, QOL and breast cancer patients.	The QOL was reassessed after 6 months to know the effect of problem focused coping strategy amongst early stage breast cancer patients comparison of 146 women (with initial stage assessment) indicating that the women who focused and keep trying to seek information about their illness experience better physical quality of life. The study made it clear that it is beneficial to seek information about symptoms. Whereas it is

		maladaptive approach to keep on focusing on the symptoms of cancer.
Al-Azri, Al- Awisi, & Moundhri, (2009).	Breast cancer patients and coping strategies .	Literature available on the impact of breast cancer diagnoses along with the strategies used by women to cope with it was reviewed to understand the associated physiological and psychological comorbities. Women diagnosed with breast cancer were found to be at risk of deterioration in an overall quality of life and multiple psychological morbidities like anxiety, depression, loneliness, fatigue, negative and suicidal thoughts, fear of death and sexual & body image problems. Strategies being often used to cope with the disease were positive cognitive restructuring, emotional expression, disease acceptance, wishful thinking, increased religious practices, family & social support, and yoga & exercise. Such knowledge is imperative for healthcare professionals and inclusion of positive ways of coping into the treatment regimen has been recommended as an important

		milestone in the palliative care,
Zhang, Gao, Wang, & Wu, (2010).	Hope, coping style, social support and breast cancer patients undergoing chemotherapy.	No any relationship between the hope level and coping style was observed, whereas hope and optimism, hope and self-reliance, and hope and palliative coping styles were positively related. On the other hand hope and the fatalistic and emotional coping styles were found to be negatively related. Hope amongst the patients with breast cancer was high and was proportional to increase in the income. During chemotherapy, patients with breast cancer adopted multiple and varying coping styles.
Karabulutla, Bilici, Meadow, Tekin, & Kantarci, (2010).	Coping strategy, anxiety, & depression and cancer patients.	The results indicated that, the prevalence of depression was in higher number of cancer patients (81.3 %) as compared to the prevalence of anxiety (61.5 %). The sample in the study mostly recruited active coping strategy and tended to avoid those stressful events which could enhance anxiety and depression. The study further revealed that social support seeking strategy was most beneficial strategy, followed by problem solving and avoiding strategy.

Subhashini, (2011).	Ways of coping and breast cancer patients.	The study on the breast cancer patients showed moderate level of coping in 52 % of the patients. The lower level of coping was observed in 20 % of the patients, whereas adequate level was observed in 28%. The results further revealed that the most frequently used coping strategy was seeking social support. Planful problem solving followed by distancing was the other important coping strategy.
Alves, Santos, & Fermandes, (2012).	Stressful situations, coping strategies and breast cancer.	The breast cancer patients exhibited stress in 66.7 % of the sample undertaken for the study. The number of stress group was found to focus mainly on problem (23.7 %) whereas in the high stress group mostly religious practices were observed (52.4 %). The role of nursing staff in training on adaptive strategy was highlighted.
Deng, Zhao, Hu, Wang, & Yu, (2014).	Coping styles, quality of life, and female breast cancer patients.	Part of the female breast cancer patients in Shanghai in 2014 mainly adopted positive coping styles. Positive coping styles seem to have had a direct relationship with QOL amongst breast cancer patients as the correlation between the two was found to be positive whereas

		negative coping of goals were found to correlate with negative coping style.
Ahadi, Delavar, & Rostami, (2014).	Copying styles, cancer patients and healthy people.	The coping strategy of cancer patients and normal healthy controls were assessed on Lazarus and Folkman''s questionnaire for comparison. The use of emotion focused coping was much higher in cancer patients. Confrontive coping, escape avoidance coping and seeking social support were used much more, whereas self-controlling, accepting responsibility, planful problem solving and positive reappraisal were hardly being used by the patients group.
Tuncay, (2014).	Ways of coping, QOL and ovarian cancer patients.	228 patients of ovarian cancer were found to use accepting emotional support and religious and the most frequently used problem focused coping strategy. Amongst the emotional focused coping self-distress wenting and behavioural disengagement was the common strategy. It was also found that problem focused coping had more relevance for spiritual and physical well-being. Whereas emotional

		focused coping were found to be inversely related with social and psychological well-being. The researcher recommended use of problem focused coping for the patients of cancer.
Liu, Shi, Yang, Rowlands, & Han , (2015).	Self-adjustment, religious coping and patients with cancer.	16 Chinese oncology patients were interviewed in depth for 0.5 - 1 hour and qualitative descriptive approach was used to analyze the results. The emerged themes were: self-adjustment including cognitive, faith and behaviour adjustment; experience of religious coping including emotional, physical and social aspects; hope and power including the hope to heal, cure and survive from cancer, or to live longer, the spiritual supporter and the helper. Thus the religious coping was found to ease stress and proved to be positive way of coping for better self-adjustment. It is recommended that the care and support system should be aware of the use of religious coping amongst oncology patients and its positive role in obtaining physiological, psychological, and spiritual comfort. Providing excellent nursing care is thus reflective of a

		holistic and multicultural environment.
Yahaya, Subramaniam, Bustam, & Tiab, (2015).	Coping strategy, Psychological & physical distress and cancer patient.	The study was conducted on 268 patients suffering from different types of cancers. It was found that emotion focused strategies were positively correlated with physical and psychological distress. It was concluded that whenever the symptom distress increased in the cancer patients they chose to use emotion focused coping. However, usually the patients employed problem focused strategy much more than the emotion focused strategy.
Maleknia, & Kahazei, (2015).	Stress, ways of coping, QOL, and breast cancer patients.	50 patients of breast cancer were studied and the results analysed Pearson‟s correlation coefficient showed a positive and significant correlation of problem focused strategy with total, symptom and functional scale of QLQ C-30. Step wise regression indicated that he functional scale was significantly correlated with problem focused coping style. At the same time emotional focused strategy was significantly but negatively correlated with functional and

		symptom dimensions of quality of life. Emotional focused coping also predicted the functional status but as a negative predictor. Problem focused coping was suggested to be better way of coping for the breast cancer patients.
Jalal, Mohamad, Ehteram, Mozafar, Hania, & Farid, (2015).	Ways of coping, QOL and cancer patients.	A mix gender group of almost equal in number was assessed on coping style as QOL to conclude that the QOL correlated positively with avoided coping style whereas it associated positively with emotional focused coping they also found that the QOL was higher among male single, high salary, educated and low age patients.
Li, Yang, Liu, &Wang, (2016).	QOL, social support, hope, resilience and bladder cancer patients.	Among the 365 patients of bladder cancer well-being was studied and it was found that to be positively correlated with social support, hope and resilience the three variables together accounted for 33.3 % of variance the well-being/ QOL.
Da Silva, Zandonade, & Amorim, (2017).	Ways of coping, anxiety and breast cancer patients.	Trait of anxiety was found to be significantly associated with problem focused strategy.
Oancea, Suciu, Timar, Papava, Raica, &	Ways of coping, anxiety, depression	Found that after one month the lung cancer diagnosis avoiding coping

Burlacu, (2018).	and lung cancer patients.	style and initial social support with increase in anxiety. His initial avoidance coping style also leads to a significant increase in the depression. In this study the adaptive coping style as a way of problem focused coping among to be the most effective coping style and avoidant style was found to be least adaptive.

The studies show a trend of emotional focus coping to be used frequently by the cancer patients. Some studies indicated that even those who usually used problem focused coping (PFC) in routine life started using PFC while suffering from cancer. Breast cancer patients seems to be good in coping as in most of studies they were reported to adopt positive ways of coping like seeking social support, planful problem solving and distancing appropriate coping has been associated with better QOL and well-being in many studies.

Many researcher have suggested that problem focused ways are better ways to cope than emotion focused coping(EFC) and they have recommended the use of PFC. However, there is no much consistency in the results obtained in the past.

Since the results of co ping style are not highly consistent and also it may require a lot of economic and human resource with longer time, it seems more appropriate to look for the ways which are simple to learn, self-administrable and can have an immediate relieving impact as required in a crises situation. **Progressive Muscle Relation or PMR** is one such established process that relieves the anxiety immediately to further reduce the effect of multiple stresses related to daily life and many other diseases. Reviews of studies of progressive muscle relaxation and cancer have been shown in table 2.8.

Table 2.8: Showing a review of studies related to PMR and cancer

Authors and year	Variables	Results
Lerman, Rimer, Blumber, Cristinzio, Engstrom, MacElwee, & O'Connor, (1990).	Coping style, cancer chemotherapy side effects, anxiety, depression, nausea associated with chemotherapy, relaxation intervention, and cancer patients.	The data was analyzed using Spearman correlations and "blunting" which is distraction-oriented coping style, was found to be significantly associated with lesser anticipatory anxiety, depression, and nausea during and after chemotherapy. On the other hand "monitoring" or information-gathering coping style was established as a poor coping style as it was found to correlate with anticipatory anxiety and more nausea before and during chemotherapy. Relaxation intervention was found to significantly reduce the nausea and vomiting. It was concluded that relaxation effectively reduces the anticipatory anxiety amongst the blunters. It was not as effective the monitors. The researchers have considered relaxation as a destruction strategy. However, anxiety being a key factor in classical conditioning module of anticipatory nausea and vomiting, the role of coping and relaxation on the pretreatment anxiety was clearly established in this study.

Molassiotis, (2000).	Breast cancer patients receiving doxorubicin & cyclophospham-ide, Progressive muscle relaxation training (PMRT), management of chemotherapy-related nausea & vomiting,	The intensity of nausea and the duration and intensity of vomiting were found to reduce as a result of PMR training. It is recommended that since the therapy is easy to learn and low cost therapy it can be used as an adjunct in the cancer treatment and nurses can impart the therapy.
Molassiotis, Yam, Yung, Chan, & Mok, (2002).	Progressive muscle relaxation training (PMRT) State-Trait Anxiety, nausea & vomiting, and breast cancer patients.	PMRT given for breast cancer patients has shown a significant improvement in the nausea and vomiting induced by chemotherapy. The PMRT has been suggested as useful adjuvant technique that can complement antiamnetics. It is further suggested that such interventions should be a part of the care plan for cancer patients who receive chemotherapy.
Yoo, Ahn, Kim, Kim, & Han, (2005).	Progressive muscle relaxation training (PMRT), guided imagery (GI), post chemotherapy nausea & vomiting (PNV), anticipatory nausea and vomiting (ANV), QOL and breast cancer patients.	A significantly lower level of anxiety, depression and hostility was recorded on PMRT and GI group in comparison to control group. These groups experienced significantly less ANV and PNV. These groups after 6 months of chemotherapy, the QOL of the PMRT and GI group was higher found to be significantly than that of the control group. Thus both PMR and GI improved the treatment associated symptoms in the breast cancer patients.

Demiralp , Oflaz, & Komurcu, (2010).	Sleep quality & fatigue, women with breast cancer and Progressive muscle relaxation training.	Progressive muscle relaxation training was given to 15 patients who had significantly improved the sleep quality and fatigue in patients with breast cancer who were undergoing adjuvant chemotherapy. Design of the study was a repeated measure quasi experiment design and multiple measures indicated the same. It was recommended that PMR should be started as chemotherapy begins so that the sleep quality can be improved and fatigue can be reduced.
Kim, & Seo, (2010).	Progressive muscle relaxation, nausea, spout, fatigue, anxiety, depression and cancer patients.	Anxiety and depression of cancer patients undergoing chemotherapy were alleviated by PMR. This has been recommended as a nursing intervention to enhance the psychological functioning amongst cancer patients.
Kashani, Babaee, Bahrami, & Valiani, (2012).	Relaxation, depression, anxiety & stress and women with breast cancer.	Depression, anxiety and stress scores in the cancer group were found to significantly improve after administering the combined medical relaxation therapy ($p < 0.05$). Relaxation therapy has been recommended as an effective care program. This included the muscular relaxation followed by a general imagery of relaxing in a beautiful garden for improvement of depression,

		anxiety and stress, amongst the malignant patients.
Isa, Moy, Abdul Razck, Zainuddin, & Zainal, (2013).	Progressive muscle relaxation training, depression, anxiety & stress and prostate cancer patients.	The module of APMR included the discussion related to anxiety and depression, focuses on breathing and brief version of PMR , „the end of relaxation Therapy" followed by a discussion on the mastery on relaxation achieved by the patients. Once trained the subjects performed relaxation daily at home for six months. The post assessment was done at four and six months. There APMR lead to significant improvements in anxiety ($p<0.001$, partial 2=0.198) and stress ($p<0.001$, partial 2=0.103). The depression did not improve significantly ($p=0.956$).
Pathak, Mahal, Kohli, & Nimbran, (2013).	Progressive muscle relaxation, State & trait, anxiety & depression, hospitalised and cancer patients receiving radiotherapy.	Depression had significantly reduced amongst the hospitalized cancer patients receiving radiotherapy, after they practiced PMR. PMR also significantly improved the quality of life of these patients. It was recommended that PMR should be included in the routine practice by nurses for the cancer patients in order to improve their quality of life.

Potthoff, Schmidt, Wiskemann, Hof, Klassen, Habermann, Beckhove, Debus, Cornelia, & Steindorf, (2013).	Resisliance training, fatigue, QOL and physical fitness molecular, immunological and inflammatory changes in breast cancer patients undergoing, adjuvant radiotherapy.	The „BEST" study is known to be the first randomized controlled trial study to compare the progressive resistance training with muscle relaxation training by taking the breast cancer patients undergoing adjuvant radiotherapy. On the basis of analysis of physiological, immunological and inflammatory parameters it is expected to contribute towards better understanding of the physiological as well as psychosocial effects along with the biological mechanisms of resistance training.
Charalambous, Giannakopoulo, Bozas, Paikkousis, (2015).	PMR, GI, anxiety & depression and breast & prostate cancer patients.	As per this study the prostate and breast cancer patients undergoing chemotherapy can benefit from PMR and GI sessions as it reduces their anxiety and depression. Anxiety and depression were both found to reduce by PMR and GI amongst prostate and breast cancer while undergoing chemotherapy. These were interpreted in terms of reducing the stress related to chemotherapy. A three weeks intervention reduced control level from 0.30± 0.25 to 0.16 ± 0.18 whereas these levels in the control group increase from 0.21± 0.22 to 0.44 ± 0.35. The difference was significant at 0.001 level. The Amylase level had

		shown the same pattern of interaction.
Zhou, Li, Li, Liu Dang, Wang, &Xin, (2015).	Anxiety, Depression, length of hospital stay, progressive muscle relaxation, Music therapy and breast cancer patients.	Progressive muscle relaxation and music therapy by cancer patients were performed twice a day for forty eight hours after radical mastectomy till before they were discharged from the hospital was found to significantly reduce and length of hospital stay. As compared to those who were not given any intervention. A significant reduction in anxiety and depression was also noted.
Charalambous, Giannakopoulou Bozas, Marcou, Kitsios, & Paikousis, (2016).	Guided Imagery (GI), Progressive Muscle Relaxation (PMR), and cancer patients.	It was found that the patients received chemotherapy had significantly improve on a cluster of symptom including fatigue, pain, HRQOL nausea and vomiting after practicing PMR and GI for four weeks. It is recommended as an intervention for the patients undergoing chemotherapy.
Kim, Na, & Hong, (2016).	Cortisol level, Stress Arousal Checklist, blood pressure, heart rate, PMRT and patients of colorectal cancer.	PMRT was found to reduce the stress assessed on cortical levels, blood pressure, stress arousal level and heart rate amongst the patients of colorectal cancer.
Koplin,Muller, Heise, Pratschke, Schwenk, &	GI, PMR and EORTC QLQ-C30 short-term QOL Gastrointestinal Quality of life Index	Neither Guided Imagery nor Progressive muscle relaxation influenced the short term QOL in this study amongst the patients of colon

Haase, (2016).	(GIQLI), and cancer patients.	cancer, the difference might be owed to the specific QOL, that is, GIQLI. The digestion may not improve.
Gupta, Kumari, & Kaur, (2016).	Progressive muscle relaxation, and cancer patients .	Physical symptoms related with chemotherapy like nausea, vomiting and pain were improved as a result of Progressive muscle relaxation in a significant number of patients. However, control group did not show any improvement. PMR was concluded to be effective in improving physical symptoms associated with chemotherapy.
Pelekasis, Matsouka, & Koumarianou, (2017).	PMR and cancer patients.	A total of 700 studies were selected from various electronic database and papers were found to be relevant. The findings indicated that PMR could improve comfort levels of cancer patients and reduce the anxiety levels as well as various side effects which are caused by chemotherapy, with an exception of vomiting. It is claimed however, that, the quality of all the included studies was extremely low. Only those studies were included that used only PMR as an intervention and the results were compared with randomized or matched control group. It was found that except vomiting the side effect of chemotherapy had

		improved, the anxiety reduced and the comfort improved as a result of PMR. Nevertheless the QOL was found to be low in all the studies included. Therefore, it is recommended that before using PMR as a standard treatment there is a need to conduct more high quality trials and test the efficiency of the technique.
Shahriari, Dehghan, Pahlavanzadeh, & Hazini, (2017).	Progressive muscle relaxation, body image, deep breathing, & QOL, and cancer patients.	Progressive muscle relaxation, guided imagery and deep diaphragmatic breathing intervention, were found to significantly improve the QOL (P<.001) and physical functioning (P<.001) amongst elderly cancer patients as compared to control group.
Tsitsi, Charalambous, Papastavrou, & Raftopoulo, (2017).	Progressive Muscle Relaxation (PMR) Guided Imagery (GI), anxiety parents of children, and cancer patients.	The levels of anxiety amongst the parents of pediatric oncology patients were found to significantly reduce by PMR and GI. The anxiety reduced in the control group also reduced with border line difference between two groups. The intervention effect size of the intervention was low to moderate. The intervention also significantly reduces the sadness and tension amongst these parents.

Relaxation intervention has been frequently reported to reduce the nausea and vomiting in the cancer patients which is a very serious issue for such patients. These side effects of chemotherapy bring many other issues like anxiety, depression, poor quality of life and well-being. PMR done and combined with guided imagery has been reported to improve the fatigue, QOL, sleep quality, anxiety ,depression, therapy related or other stresses, length of hospital stay and physiological parameter like arousal, heart rate and blood pressure among the patients of cancer. On depression some studies have reported contradictory results as PMR did not have any positive effects on depression. Radiotherapy associated effects were also found to reduce by PMR practice. Most of the studies have reported PMR to be highly beneficial, and recommended that it should be integrated part of cancer treatment. Many have suggested that nurses can be trained to give PMR and GI to such patients.

With this background it seems highly relevant to study these variables in relation to cancer in India. Therefore the specific problem and hypotheses were framed, which have been discussed in the next chapter.

CHAPTER III

PROBLEM AND HYPOTHESES

Cancer being amongst the top 10 causes of death in the nation, rank 2nd 2.25 million cancer cases are estimated to exist in India at any given point of time. According to (Khatoon, 2012) each year detects about 10 lakh patients as per in other estimates more than 7 lakh new cases are detected while 3 lakhs would die by cancer each year. As per the population based registry (NCRP) it is evident that oral cavity, esophagus, stomach and lung cancer are the major site of cancer amongst men. Women suffer from oral cavity, breast cancer and cervix cancer. More than 50% of the total cancer mortality in India accounts to the lung and oral cavity cancer amongst male and breast cancer and cervix cancer amongst female. The estimate of WHO use of tobacco contributing to 90% of oral cancer in south-east Asia, which also a leading cause of lung and oral cavity cancer in India (Rao, Gupta &Agarwal,2002). The lung cancer, prostate cancer, breast cancer, colon cancer and the pancreatic cancer are five leading cancer causing death (Kochanek, XU, & Murphy, 2011).

Cancer is very major chronic health concerned around the global taking one life in every 90 seconds. In India also it is one of the 10 reasons of mortality. Medically, this covers more than 250 types for which cancer is a general term. The factors which influence the development of cancer include genetic link (Claus, Risch, & Thompson, 1993), ethnicity (Meyerowitz, Richardson, Hudson, & Leedham, 1998), life style factors (Brownson et al., 1993; Rao, Gupta, & Agarwal, 2002; Calle, Miracle-McMahill, Thun, & Heath, 1994), diet (Meyerhardt et al., 2007; Protta, Charrel, & Cappa, 1989; Slattery, Boucher, Can, Pooter, & Ma,1998; Toniolo, Ribloi, Shekelle, Rosspf, & Stemler, 1991; Zhang et.at.,1999;), sun exposure (Brownson et al., 1993; Koh et al,1997), sexual behavior (Brownsonet et al. 1993), excessive alcohol use (Heuch, Kvale, Jacobson & Bjelke, 1983), stress (Delahanty& Baum, 2001; Grossarth, Bastisams, Kanazin, Scimdt & Vetter, 1992; McKenna, Zevon, Corn, & Round, 1999; Jacobs & Charles, 1980) and personality (Dattore, Shontz, & Coyene, 1980; Persky, Kemthorne-Rawson, & Shekelle, 1987; Roberts, Newcomb, Trentham-

Dietz, & Storer, 1996;Shaffer, Graves, Swank, & Person, 1987). The disease has been known to company many psychiatric and non-psychiatric issues. Leads to severe anxiety, a perceived loss of control, cognitive impairment including confusing or disorientation. Depression can be observed in the form of multiple symptoms i.e. sleep disturbing, crying, dejection, misery, suicidal ideation, hopelessness and worthlessness etc. In other words at a psychological level cancer is known to enhance the stress in its multiple forms. Stress has been clearly known to weaken the immune system; thereby decreasing the body potential to deduct and kill the abnormal cancer cell (Delahanty & Baum, 2001). In this way the stress accompanied by any type of cancer heightens the difficulties in its treatment; thus calling for positive coping.

Not only this, the given medication, chemotherapy and radiotherapy bring in their own side effect (Bovbjerg, 1990; Burish, Meyerowitz, Carey, & Morrow, 1987; Jacobsen, 1993). These may include the anxiety and fear of treatment i.e. nausea, vomiting, loss of appetite, loss of hair and fatigue etc. which further strengthen the need of improvement in coping. As discussed in chapter 1 and 2 all this tends to reduce the hope, quality of life and subjective well-being of cancer patients. The factors like hospital anxiety, resilience and hope are also expected to influence the quality of life and well-being of cancer patients (Ha, Jung, & Choi, 2014; Li, Lin, Liang, Hu, Lan, Liang, Zeng, Wang, & Fu, 2017).

It is very clear from the last two chapters that cancer is a serious concerns it brings many more problems with it e.g. creating anxiety, depression and a variety of maladjustment. The disease itself is shocking and its acceptance is difficult for both the patient and the family. The treatment also brings along a lot of serious side effects and it may become difficult to take the treatment easy, leading to further deterioration in one"s mental state. All this also leads to a huge financial cost and the family burden in terms of energy and the time involved in the treatment. There is every possibility that the reduced physical and psychological health would lead to reduced positive mental health states in a subjects suffering from cancer. Therefore, an active coping is required to deal with the problems related with cancer. All this makes it necessary to study the ways of coping from three viewpoints. (1) As adapted by the cancer patients. (2) As related to one"s mental health, and (3) to understand these ways to prepare specific intervention programs. There are studies in the literature indicating that positivity, social support, distancing etc. lead to less emotional problems (Dunkel- Schetter et al., 1992; Stanton & Snider, 1993). But the studies in this and the above discussed contexts are still not sufficient to conclude and decide about the interventions that can be utilized. Particularly, the Indian studies in this area seem to be very less. Therefore, it would carry wide implications for the cancer patients if their coping style and subjective well-being, hope, resilience are understood and interpreted with the above aims in mind. However, regarding the 3rd viewpoint instead of designing any intervention strategies, progressive muscular relaxation would be taken up. Relaxation includes deep and brief methods. Progressive muscular deep relaxation is a method in which the individual is learns on what and how „it feels like" when the muscles are relaxed over while these are tense. This is a method of making a direct comparison and learning by practice, which is expected to relieve an individual from all kinds of anxiety, depression, fatigue etc. Once learnt, individuals can self-administer it. Therefore, there is no need of any trained psychotherapist. Keeping all this in mind the following problem was formulated. Therefore it is necessary to understand the effect of cancer on positive mental health along with research of the ways of enhancing the positive mental health. Knows about the ways of coping that have a positive influence will help in sensitizes the patient of future and knows the effect of PMR will also be a reflection upon designing the required intervention. So the following problem was formulated.

Problem:

To study the positive mental health e.g. coping styles, subjective well-being, quality of life, resilience and hope amongst the patients of cancer and the impact of progressive muscular relaxation on these variables.

Objectives

1. To assess and compare the ways of coping, subjective well-being, quality of life, resilience & hope among the patients of different types of cancer with normal healthy controls.

2. To study the correlation of coping style with subjective well-being, quality of life, resilience & hope in the cancer patients.

3. To study the impact of progressive muscle relaxation on quality of life, subjective well-being , quality of life, resilience, hope, fatigue and hospital anxiety on patients suffering from different types of cancers.

Hypotheses

1. The quality of life, subjective well- being, hope and resilience in all type of cancer patients would be lesser than the normal healthy controls.

2. Higher the problem focused coping higher would be the quality of life, subjective well-being, hope and resilience in both the patients and the healthy controls.

3. Progressive muscle relaxation would enhance the quality of life, subjective well- being, resilience and hope.

4. Progressive muscle relaxation would reduce the fatigue and hospital anxiety.

CHAPTER-IV

METHODOLOGY

Introduction in chapter 1 highlighted that the prevalence of various type of cancer is a serious disease burden around the globe. India also suffers from high prevalence and incidence of cancer and the consequent psychological and physiological/ biological comorbities. Therefore, it is important to look for simple interventions for the care of oncology patients and reduce the disease burden on patient, family, health sector and the nation. A careful look at chapter 2 shows that studies in India are very less. So the study was conducted with a major aim to asses some of the psychological accompaniment of cancer on Indian oncology patients and investigate if PMR can help in doing away with some of these disturbance. To verify the hypotheses formed in chapter 3 following design were used.

Design

In phase I

The study was conducted in two phases. In phase 1,a multi-groups design was employed to assess the patients on the various positive mental health indicators amongst four types of cancer. Breast, cervix, lung and prostate cancer were selected because of relatively higher prevalence.

Group 1	**Group 2**	**Group 3**	**Group 4**	**Group 5**
Breast cancer patients	Cervix cancer patients	Lung cancer patients	Prostate cancer patients	Normal healthy controls

n=50, N=250

In phase II, a pre-post study on 40 cancer patients undergoing treatment, was conducted to assess the impact of Progressive muscular relaxation.

Sample

200 patients of cancer, 50 each suffering from lung, breast, cervix and prostate cancer were selected from PGIMS, Rohtak and from other nearby places on the basis of availability and consent of the participants. At the later stage, the patients were also taken from Rajiv Gandhi cancer hospital by contacting them in the OPD. These patients were placed in Rohtak, Jhajjar and nearby places. The age range was restricted to 30 –50 years. An effort was made to equate the groups (as much as possible) with respect to various socio demographic variables e.g. socio economic status, occupation, rural - urban background and stage of cancer etc. as much as possible. However, the mode of treatment could be any, i.e., chemotherapy, radiotherapy or both. A parallel control group of normal and healthy subjects were selected in the same way. Subjects at the terminal stage were not included in the study. Completely illiterate subjects were also not included in the study.

Tools

1. **EORTC QLQ-C30. (version 3)**

The European organization for research and treatment of cancer quality of life questionnaire, EORTC QLQ-C30. Questionnaire usually written as EORTC QLQ-C30 is a 30 item questionnaire which is highly cancer specific (Aaronson, Ahmedzai, & Bergman,1993). The present questionnaire QLQ C30 was designed to cover multiple aspects and dimensions of QOL as embedded in the concept.

This multi-dimensional tool has been structured with simplicity to be brief and easy; thus being highly appropriate for self-administration. Its empirically validated applicability across a wide range of cultural settings is an inbuilt strength. The tool is therefore, apt and fit for use in research or clinical trials of cancer therapy/ies. This questionnaire is very specific with focused questions that are designed to assess oncology relevant aspects of quality of life; thus being modular and highly relevant in its applicability to a wide range of all types of cancer patients.

QLQ C-30 is comprehensive measuring symptom QOL, functional QOL, and global health status by answering the given 30 items. These are scored on four point scale ranging from "not at all" to "very much". It also measures the QOL overall along with the earlier mentioned three more aspects of functional status, symptom status and global health status. Global health status measures the subjective experience and perception of individual"s overall quality of life in concern to the disease. However, the questions have been designed in such a manner that it can be performed on normal healthy controls also and most of the studies have used it in the past. This way, QLQ C-30 has an added advantage of being research friendly by enabling the researchers to make a comparison of the QOL of cancer patients with healthy controls.

On all the dimensions the range of scores can vary between 0-100. On functional scale and global health scales higher scores represent a better or healthier level of functioning and higher global QOL respectively. On symptom scale, the higher score indicates lower QOL or higher symptomology.

2. FACT-G

The Functional assessment of cancer general version (FACT-G version 4) was developed by David Cella (1997) by a continuous assessment of the patients who were undergoing the clinical trial for cancer therapy: assess the well-being of cancer patients in a quantitative way. After 3 reviews, the present version has subscales covering four dimensions i.e. physical well-being, social/family well-being, emotional well-being and functional well-being. 27 Items in the present scale for are rated from 0-4. The five responses varied from „not at all" to "very much". The tool is highly appropriate for application patients with any type of cancer, and even the extensions the tool is very specific but has also been validated for use in other chronic illness condition like HIV/AIDS; Parkinson's disease; multiple sclerosis; rheumatoid arthritis the best feature is that it can be used for the general population too. Questions measure the respondents" health state over last 7 days. The initial version had 33 items and was developed over the hard work of 6 years between 1987 & 93. The tool has been designed to enhance the clarity and precision of assessment. Latest version is a simple version as the revisions were focused on item reduction, simplification and reward. The tool has already being translated in more than 60 languages and is being used worldwide.

Reliability of FACT-G was assessed by calculating cronbach alpha found to be more than .90 for the application and individual level and more than .70 for application at group level. The reliability of the total FACT-G and its individual subscales was calculated by using cronbach alpha.

Convergent validity was found to be high when tested against Functional Living Index – Cancer, Brief Profile of Mood States, the Taylor Manifest Anxiety Scale, and patient-reported ECOG Performance Status. Divergent validity was also calculated by using the Marlowe-Crowne social desirability scale. Divergent validity was also calculated for this the correlation between different construct were calculated and were found to be low.

Scoring is done by summing the score on all subscales. The scoring on physical and emotional well-being was in reverse order. In other words higher the score lower the physical and emotional well-being. On the other hand, for the other two dimensions of functional well-being and social & family well-being relationship is direct; higher the score higher the well-being.

3. **Multidimensional Fatigue Inventory (MFI)**

The MFI was constructed by Smets, Garssen, & Bonke, (1995). It is a twenty items self-report instrument that measures fatigue. It five dimensions consisting of four items each are mental fatigue, general fatigue, physical fatigue, reduced activity and reduced motivation. The scale is composed of both positively and negatively worded statements, in equal number of check any probable response bias. The respondent indicates the extent to which the particular statement applies to the respondent. The five point scale of response varies from "Yes, that is true" and "No, that is not true."

There are five scales in MFI-20 which have been structured by considering various modes of expressing the fatigue. In this the scale measures general fatigue, physical fatigue, mental fatigue, reduced activity and reduced motivation. General fatigue pertains to everyday functioning while physical fatigue is a major measure of somatic symptoms. The reduced desire or drive to initiate the required activities has been called as reduced motivation while the actual reduction in carrying out the activities has been called as reduced activity. Cognition reduction, including the power of concentration is called mental fatigue.

4. Hospital Anxiety and Depression Scale (HADS)

The Hospital Anxiety and Depression Scale (HADS) were developed in 1983 by Zigmond and Snaith. The scale consists of 14 items. Each question is responded on four point scales. Seven of these questions are meant to address anxiety, whereas am equal number is designed to assess depression. These have been designed particularly for the cancer patients.

The test is a self-assessment scale. It was developed to assess depression, anxiety and emotional distress amongst patients under treatment for various clinical problems (Zigmond & Snaith 1983), but it was prepared as a clinical diagnostic tool (Whelan-Goodinson, Ponsford, & Schonberger, 2009). Initially, the contained eight items in it, that was related to depression and other eight were pertaining to anxiety which were later reduced to seven for each measures. Correlations ranged between +0.60 & +0.30, with a significance of $p<0.02$. The correlations of anxiety ranged between +0.76 & +0.41 ($p<0.01$). The responses are scored on a scale of 0-3 where 3 indicates higher symptom frequencies (Whelan-Goodinson et al., 2009). In this way the scores for each subscale (anxiety and depression) fall under a possible range of 0 to 21.These score are categorized as severe: 15-21, moderate: 11-14, mild: 8-10, normal: 0-7. Scores for the entire scale would thus range from 0 to 42. The higher scores is indicative of higher distress. Since the focus is on subjective assessments, the patients are asked to *"fill it completely in order to reflect how they have been feeling during the past week"* (Zigmond & Snaith, 1983), before they start working on the given Performa.

5. The Adult Hope Scale

The adult hope scale (ADHS) was constructed by Snyder, Irving, & Anderson in 1991.According to him Adult hope scale *„is a measure of individual"s intended succession in congruence to the identified goals"*. In other words hope is a measure of the „determination of an individual to achieve the goal". The present scale consists is a small but all inclusive type of measure with 12 items. These items are to be responded on an 8 point Likert scale of: Definitely true, Mostly true, Somewhat true, Slightly true, Slightly false, Somewhat false, Mostly false and Definitely false.

The questionnaire is easy self-report measure on which 4 of the 12 given items tap agency thoughts, 4 tap the pathways thoughts and rest of the 4 are meant for inclusion in hope total. The scale thus gives three types of scores, that is, agency score, pathways score and a total hope score that is obtained by summing the scores on the items meant to assess the agency and pathway components. Total hope scale scores, in this way can vary between 8- 64 as the minimum and maximum limits. Accordingly, agency and pathway scores may vary between 4-32 as the lower and the upper limits. The interpretation of on all the sub scales is direct. In other words higher the scores higher the hope (Snyder et al, 1991).

The Adult hope scale has very high levels of reliability. The Cronbach alphas were between .74 to .84 for overall hope, .71 to .76 for agency thoughts and .63 to .80 for pathway thoughts. This was all done against student and clinical population and samples. Test-retest reliability was also measured Snyder (1991). This was found to be .80 or above for time gap taken up to 10 weeks for normal student population only.

The convergent and discriminant validity of the scale were highly supported when tested. Validity of the scale was assessed with the help of correlation with scores on the Life orientation test (Scheier & Carver, 1985). This correlation was found to be positive. With the Hopelessness Scale by Beck, Weissman, Lester, & Trexler, (1974) this scale was found to be negatively correlated while it did not correlate when tested against Self Consciousness Scale by Fenigstein, Scheier & Buss (1975).

6. **Resilience Scale**

Wagnild and Young (1993) prepared Resilience scale consisting of 26 items. The responses on seven point scale vary from strongly disagree, to disagree. The total possible score thus ranges from 26 to 182 ranges with higher scores reflecting higher resilience. This scale is applicable on a wide range of population covering all ages, socio economic status and educational background etc. The present revised version was been given in 2009, comprising 14 items. **Reliability,** Cronbach"s alpha ranges from .87 to .95.

According to Wagnild and Young (1993), the items of the scale were selected to reflect five interrelated elements of resilience. First is the *existential aloneness* that pertains to recognition that the life path of each individual is different and unique. Second is *meaningfulness* indicating that life has some relevant goal and is purposeful. *Self-reliance* measure the extent of how much one can depend on myself i.e. a perspective about the belief and trust in one's abilities. *Perseverance* is an art of continuing or being glued to. In other words persistence to carry on during adversity is the fourth kind of inclusion and measurement. *Equanimity* is the last component which pertains to a balanced outlook of one's life and experiences. All the five components were included while constructing this scale, though the scale gives a single score on resilience.

The internal consistency was also assessed by the developers before publishing and later again Wagnild (2010). The cronbach alpha were found to be .91 and .93 respectively the scale has very wide applicability and has translated in Russian (Aroian, Schappler-Morris, Neary, Spitzer, & Tran, 1997), Spanish (Heilemann, Lee, & Kury, 2003), Nigerian (Abiola & Udofia, 2011), Swedish (Nygeren, Aléx, Jonsén, Gustafson, Norberg, & Lundman, 2005) and Japanese (Nishi, Uehara, Kondo,& Matsuoka, 2010). Thus the scale has a wide applicability around the globe.

7. Ways of Coping (Revised).

Ways of Coping (Revised) of coping four point scales was developed by Folkman and Lazarus (1980). It consists of 66 items. The ways of coping scale is a measure to identify the pattern of thoughts and behaviour used by an individual in a specific stressful situation. This scale was particularly chosen because the study refers to cancer patients and „dealing with cancer" is a specific situation. This scale across the coping process and not the coping disposition or the coping style this definition has four key features: it is process-oriented; it speaks of management rather than mastery; it makes no prior judgment about the quality of coping processes; and it implies a stress-based distinction between coping and automatic adaptive behaviours.

It measures mainly the problem focused coping and emotional focused coping. Problem focused coping include planful problem solving, confrontive coping, and seeking social support. While emotional focused coping comprises of positive reappraisal, distancing, accepting responsibility, self-controlling and escape avoidance emotional focused coping ways of coping pertain to how one can manage one"s emotional response to everyday pressures and stressors, while the focus in problem focus strategies remain upon the changing aspects of the daily surroundings and along with the relationship of individual. When an individual adopts the strategy by focusing or working upon changing aspects of the environment as well as individual relationship with the environment it is called problem focused ways of coping. Emotional Focus Coping, on the other hand focuses upon how one manages one"s emotions and how one responds to the stressor (Folkman and Lazarus, 1980; Lazarus 1993). In this way there are total 8 scales. There are four possible responses, 0,1,2,3 0stipulates "does not apply", 1 stipulates "used somewhat", 2 stipulates "used quite a bit" and 3 stipulates "used a great deal". The score obtained in this way are totaled to get the raw score. The higher the raw score higher is the strategy used by the patients. The problem solving includes items pertaining to:

- **Confronting coping** pertains to measurement of aggressive effort to alter the situation". This scale is also suggestive of the degree of risk taking and hostility used to cope up by the individual.
- **Seeking social support** pertains to the use of tangible support, seeking informational support and the emotional support.
- **Planful problem solving** means deliberate problem focused efforts steps taken by the subject to change the particular as situation, couples with an analytic approach to move towards solution of problem.

The emotion focused coping measures include the following:

- **Positive reappraisal** this is an effort to create positive meaning by focusing on individual personal growth. A religious dimension has also been included in it.

- **Distancing**is a measure of made by individual cognitive effort to detach one in order to minimize the significance of given situation.
- **Self-controlling** is deliberate effort to regulate one"s feelings and behavioural actions.
- **Accepting responsibility** is acknowledging one"s own role in the problem with special reference to the concomitant theme of „trying to put things right".
- **Escape avoidance** is desired way of cognitive and behavioural efforts used to escape or avoid the particular problem. The items on this scale contrast with those on the distancing scale that suggest detachment.

Reliability for the eight scale estimated with Cronbach"s coefficient alpha, is as follows .70 for Conforntive Coping,.61 for Distancing, .70 for Self –controlling, .76 for Seeking social support, .66 for Accepting Responsibility, .68 for Planful Problem Solving, .79 for Positive Reappraisal. The validity lies between 0.17 and 0.47.

Procedure

First of all, the tools were translated in Hindi. For translation the researcher translated the tools in simple Hindi and then gave it to four judges from psychology, expert of Hindi & two from English. The comments were analyzed to make the required changes if the judges reported any sentence to be vague or ambiguous. Now one professional in Hindi with command on English and another professional in English with a command in Hindi were given these questioner for back translation on the basis of this the questioner were finalized. Permission from the authorities of PGIMS, Rohtak was taken and the patients were contacted in the O.P.D as well as in the wards. Good rapport was built with the patients and they were made willing for filling up of the questionnaire. For developing a rapport, the patients were informed of the purpose and implication of the study. This helped in motivating the patients the patients co-operate even if they were in pain. An informed consent was taken and confidentiality was assured. The subjects were properly instructed and the tools were filled on one to one bases. After filling up all the tools, scoring and analyses was performed. In 2nd phase of the study subjects having poor quality of life, subjective well-being, hope and resilience, were selected. Those having lower level, preferably on the all the 4 variables were selected and 10 sessions of progressive muscle relaxation were given on the alternate days. Now the post assessment was done. The patients were informed about the purpose of giving them progressive muscle relaxation. However, they were not told that they will have a positive effect. They were just told that this is a tryout to know if PMR will affect the cancer patients in any way. After this they were informed that they will be made to listen to a CD in which they will be asked to tense and relax certain set of muscle in a sequence. They were told to follow the instructions sincerely and note the difference between the state when the muscles were tense and relaxed. They were explained and demonstrated about the posture of the muscle to be taken while turning and relaxing them. A pre-recorded set of imagery was also presented through CD in continuation with the muscle relaxation. As recommended by Batra, (2008) a general imagery pertaining to enjoying with family / friends around the lake.

In this way 15 sessions were given to the 10 patients in each group of cancer on alternate day. After two days of the test session post assessment was done and the scores were put to analyses. The obtained results in both phases of study have been discussed in the next chapter.

CHAPTER-V

RESULTS AND DISCUSSION

The purpose of present work was to assess and understand the quality of life, subjective well-being, hope and resilience amongst cancer patients; to understand their ways of coping; and to check if PMR can help the cancer patients. For this various objectives and hypotheses were formulated as given in chapter 3. To test these hypotheses, present study was conducted in two phases. Multi group design was used in the first phase of study. The second phase was a pre-post study to understand the effect of PMR on psychological state of cancer patients by considering the variables of QOL, well-being, hope, resilience, fatigue and hospital anxiety & depression. After assessing the cancer patients on various measures and collecting the data, obtained scores were tabulated and analyzed by using statistical package for the social sciences (SPSS-20).

First hypothesis predicted that the quality of life, health related well-being, hope and resilience in various types of cancer patients would be poorer than the normal healthy control groups. A multi-group design in phase one was employed by selecting five groups i.e. breast, cervix, lungs & prostate cancer groups and a control group of 50 patients each. The means of these groups on various dimensions have been shown in table 5.1.

Table 5.1: Showing the means of various cancer groups and control group on QOL, well-being (FACT-G), hope and resilience.

Cancer types / Dimensions	Breast cancer	Cervix cancer	Lungs cancer	Prostate cancer	Control group
QOL	167.68	161.79	161.12	159.75	175.93
Well-being(Fact G)	46.28	48.44	47.6	50.88	47.00
Hope	46.1	41.96	45.6	44.96	54.64
Resilience	140.62	131.3	141.92	129.38	143.42

The mean values indicate that there was a *negative impact of cancer on quality of life, hope and resilience,* as these were found to be lower in all of the cancer patient groups than the control group. However, the well-being (FACT-G) of prostate cancer group was highest, while other groups were more or less equal to control subjects and well-being.

FACT-G means which indicate the scores on well-being are not showing any consistent trend. This is because of the fact that the scoring of two out of four subscales is in reverse order. Therefore, the total mean will be ignored for analysis while considering the scores on all four subscales separately for analysis as is discussed in the following sections.

The study being a multi-group design, one way ANOVA was applied to all the mean scores. The following table shows obtained F value on various variables.

Table 5.2: Showing the F values of different variables after applying one way ANOVA to all five groups (Breast, cervix, lung & prostate cancer, and control group).

Variable	F Values	Level of significance
QLQ-C30	9.347	.000
Well-being (FACT-G)	2.17	.073
Hope	17.572	.000
Resilience	3.569	.008

Table 5.2 indicates that the F values for hope, resilience and quality of life were found to be significant whereas F value for Fact–G total well-being was not significant. The significant values do not present a clear picture to indicate that which of the group means are significantly different at what level from each other. So the post hoc analysis was employed and DRT was used. Following section is the description and discussion of the F values and DRTs employed to study the significance of difference in these variables amongst cancer patients as compared to normal healthy controls.

QOL of cancer patients was assessed on EROTC QLQ C-30 version 3. To understand the quality of life amongst cancer patients, means of all four types of cancer patients and control group on overall quality of life, functional status, symptom status and global health status were calculated. The overall means of patients on quality of life are much lower than the normal subjects and the quality of life amongst cancer patients seems to have reduced.

To understand this negative impact on QOL in depth, One Way ANOVA was applied on various dimensions of QOL and the results have been shown in table 5.3.

Table 5.3: Showing the F values on various dimensions of quality of life and overall quality of life after applying one way ANOVA on all the five groups.

Variable	F value	Level of significance
Quality of life (Total)	5.798	.000
Functional scale	10.966	.000
Symptom scale	14.874	.000
Global health status	12.695	.000

Significant F values for all the dimensions of quality of life indicate that overall quality of life, functional scale, symptom scale and global health status scores differed significantly amongst the four groups of cancer and control group. Therefore, to understand the specific differences in various groups of cancer, post hoc DRT was applied (Table 5.4).

Table 5.4: Showing the means of various groups and summaries of DRTs applied to the scores on functional scale, symptom scale, global health status and total overall quality of life amongst all types of cancer groups and healthy controls.

Groups and means / Dimensions	Prostate cancer	Lungs cancer	Cervix cancer	Breast cancer	Control group
Total quality of life	159.75	161.12	161.79	167.68	175.93
Functional scale	**Cervix cancer**	**Prostate cancer**	**Breast cancer**	**Lungs cancer**	**Control group**
	63.95	69.24	72.2	72.2	81.95
Symptom scale	**Control group**	**Breast cancer**	**Lungs cancer**	**Prostate cancer**	**Cervix cancer**
	14.97	29.79	29.89	35.17	38
Global health status	**Prostate cancer**	**Lungs cancer**	**Cervix cancer**	**Breast cancer**	**Control group**
	55.3	59	59.83	65.66	79

It can be seen from table 5.4 that mean value of control group was 175.93 which is significantly higher than all cancer groups on **total QOL**. Higher mean values indicate better quality of life. Thus QOL of all types of cancer groups selected in this study was significantly worse than healthy normal control group. However, there is no significant difference in quality of life among different cancer groups. So the quality of life of lungs, breast, prostate and cervix cancer group was found to be equally worse.

Table 5.4 further indicates that the mean value of control group in the quality of life **functional scale** was 81.95 which is higher than all groups of cancer patients. Higher mean scores represent a higher or better quality of life on functional status. Thus the quality of life was found to be significantly lower in all types of cancer patients participating in the study than normal healthy people. The summaries of DRT in the above table 5.4 also indicate that, functional status of quality of life was found to be worst in cervix cancer group, as the cervix cancer group was significantly poor from breast and lung cancer group too. Quality of life of cervix cancer patients was significantly worse than healthy women on functional status, and than lung & breast cancer patients. However, there is no significant difference amongst lung, breast and prostate cancer groups. Also no significant difference existed between prostate, lung and breast cancer groups.

Regarding **symptom scale** QOL, as indicated in table 5.4, the mean value of control group was 14.97 which is lower than all groups of cancer patients. Lower mean scores indicate fewer problems i.e. lower the score better the quality of life on symptom status. Higher score of symptom scale represents a high level of symptomatology/ problems. Thus the quality of life on symptom status was found to be significantly lower in all types of cancer patients taken in this study than normal healthy controls. In other words the symptoms were higher in the cancer patients. The summary of DRT in the above table 5.4 further indicates that quality of life symptom status was found to be lowest in cervix cancer group and least worse in the breast cancer group. There is no significant difference between prostate and cervix cancer groups but the prostate cancer group mean differed significantly from breast and lungs cancer groups. There is no significant difference amongst breast, lungs and prostate cancer groups. To conclude, each type of cancer led to a significant reduction in symptom status QOL and the cervix cancer patients were affected the most; thus being the worst hit on quality of life symptom scale by cancer.

As indicated in table 5.4, **global health status QOL** scores show that the mean value of control group is 79 which is significantly higher than the mean scores of all other cancer groups. Higher mean scores represent better quality of life. Global health score of breast cancer group is significantly less affected than prostate cancer groups, while the maximum worsening can be seen in case of prostate cancer group which also differed significantly from breast cancer. However, no significant differences existed between breast, cervix and lungs cancer groups. Similarly no significant differences existed between prostate, lungs and cervix cancer groups.

Summarily it is interesting to note that in spite of reverse scoring on symptomatology, the total QOL was significantly poor in each group of cancer patients. Global health status refers to the perception of quality of life assessed by asking only two direct questions pertaining to overall feelings of quality of life, on which prostate cancer patients were the worst hit and breast cancer patients were significantly better than prostate cancer patients, though significantly poor than controls. The functional status QOL was a worst hit in case of cervix cancer patients and symptom status QOL was also found to be the worst in the cervix cancer patients, which were also significantly worse than breast cancer patients. It would not be erroneous to say that breast cancer patients were better than other groups on QOL, because their perception was significantly less poor on QOL global health status and significantly low on symptomatology than some or the other groups of cancer. Therefore, in spite of differences in different types of cancer on various dimensions of QOL, the first hypothesis predicting the quality of life, subjective well-being, hope and resilience in all types of cancer patients would be lesser than normal healthy controls has proved for QOL as total QOL was significantly lower amongst all types of cancer under taken.

In the past researches, Kristen & GerdInger, (2014), found that the QOL of the patients of cancer was significantly lower than the people who never experienced cancer. Greater proportion of cervix cancer patients had poor overall quality of life. The quality of life of cancer patients was found to be poor in cervix cancer patients in many studies (Dahiya et al., 2016; Khalil et al., 2015; Li et al., 2017; Swangvaree & Kosiyatrasul, 2010) and also in cervix cancer survivors (Torkzahrani et al., 2013). In fact amongst cervix cancer patients and amongst the cervix cancer survivors quality of life was better. It was negatively associated with symptomatology while it was positively associated with economic and social conditions of the patients. Cervix cancer patients reported to generally have a decent global quality of life that was equivalent with healthy controls. But they experienced relatively lower sexual functioning and enjoyment. Their satisfaction with their body image was also poor than the healthy controls (Khalil et al., 2015).

The quality of life amongst lung cancer patients was poor than the healthy population (Polanski et al., 2016; Pradhan et al., 2015). In the same way quality of life was poor amongst the lung cancer patients in some other studies also (Akin et al., 2010; Benbrahim et al., 2016; Henoch et al., 2007; Polanski et al., 2016; Montazeri et al., 2001) and many more, as discussed in second chapter. Yang et al., (2012), found that the survivors of lung cancer suffered from a substantial symptom burden. They also recommended that lung cancer survivors must be exposed to the interventions to improve the health related quality of life. Montazeri (2001) found in his study that perception of symptoms and stress play an important role. Higher the perception of symptoms and stress, lower is the quality of life.

In the same way the quality of life among breast cancer patients was found to be poor in various studies (Ristevska-Dimitrovska et al., 2015; Ahmed, et al., 2016; Ha, et al., 2014). In one study Deng et al., (2017) also found that higher resilience was correlated with better quality of life among the breast cancer patients. Prostate cancer patients showed poor quality of life in studies conducted by Engl et al., (2017) and Vashistha et al., (2016).

Chean et al., (2016) found that the emotional and social functioning were significantly better amongst the patients of breast cancer having undergone three cycles of chemotherapy than those who were not yet given the chemotherapy. On the other hand symptoms related QOL had become much poorer particularly for the significant appetite loss and significant increase in nausea and vomiting.

Ivanauskiene, (2010) conducted a study on breast cancer patients. They found that the QOL amongst these patients was though lower than the population living without cancer, yet this QOL was pretty good. These patients were poor on fatigue and sleep. Most important factors influencing the general HRQOL were fatigue and pain. They also found that women at the terminal stage were poor on QOL; particularly in terms of social activity than the women diagnosed immediately. The study also claimed that this fairly QOL was poor than the corresponding population in the other countries. This study was conducted on 284 patients in Lithuania (Europe). In an Indian study by Pandey et al., (2015), the same version of questionnaire that is EROTC QOL C-30 was used to assess the quality of life of cancer patients. They found that QOL of cancer patients was influenced by factors like site of cancer, type of cancer and the time elapsed after onset of cancer. They also found that the overall quality of life of cancer patients was significantly correlated with its own various dimensions, e.g., physical, cognitive, emotional, social role functioning and the symptoms like loss of appetite, nausea, pain, fatigue and dyspnea etc. Even the financial problems were found to be correlated with overall quality of life.

It is interesting to note that Kristen (2014) indicated in his study that there is evidence showing the difference in QOL of the patients in different countries. Accordingly it seems relevant to conduct such a study in India to cater to the needs of cancer patients in the nation.

The above studies show that earlier literature is indicative of lower or poor quality of life amongst all type of cancer patients like in the present piece of research on cervix, breast, lung and prostate cancer. In the above studies, previous researchers have either conducted the studies by taking only one type of cancer, or they have taken only one group of cancer with variety of cancers in it. Therefore, present researcher was unable to find the studies in which various types of cancer have been compared to understand how these differ from each other. So which type of cancer has been a worst or least hit quality of life of patients, could not be compared with the past studies. However, these findings are clearly indicating that prostate cancer seems to bring more deterioration amongst men and cervix cancer seems to bring more deterioration of QOL amongst women. These are important findings, which need to be verified further, along with an attempt to find the reasons. It is also suggested „that type specific interventions" should be designed.

However, higher fatality in the cervix cancer explains the findings of this study on cervix cancer. Breast cancer has replaced cervix cancer as leading cause of cancer deaths amongst women in India. In 2013, the number of women who died due to cervical cancer was 40985 while it was 47,587 for breast cancer patients (https://indianexpress.com/article/india/india-others/breast-cancer-top-killer-among-women-lung-cancer-among-men-in-india/, retrievedon 24/8/2018). It is notable that the prevalence of breast cancer is very high than cervix cancer.

Health related well-being (FACT- G):

FACT-G is also a cancer specific questionnaire and measures health related quality of life in terms of**well-being**in four domains i.e. physical, social & family, emotional and functional well-being.

As already discussed, F value on total score was insignificant. This fact was ignored in view of the fact the two of the four scale have reveres scoring Therefore, the analysis of Fact G was done on all the four subscale separately and the obtained means have been shown in Table 5.5.

Table 5.5: Showing the meansof cancer patients and normal controls on the subscalesof FACT- G.

Cancer groups / FACT-G Dimensions	Breast cancer	Cervix cancer	Lungs cancer	Prostate cancer	Control group
Total	46.28	48.44	47.6	50.88	47
Physical well being	8.22	11.62	9.92	11.78	3.62
Social and family well being	17.68	16.9	18.76	17.68	16.66
Emotional well being	5.9	7.88	5.40	7.72	6.16
Functional well being	14.56	12.14	13.88	13.76	20.56

The meaning of score and its indicators has been discussed while discussing the DRT results. However, since the means are differing, one way ANOVA was applied. The following table shows the F values when one way ANOVA was applied to all the four dimensions of FACT-G.

Table 5.6 indicates that F values for physical well-being, emotional well-being and functional well-being were significant and for social & family well-being F value was not significant. This indicates that physical, emotional and functional well-being differed significantly amongst the four groups of cancer and the control group.

Table 5.6: Showing the F values on various dimensions of FACT-Gafter applying one way ANOVA on all the five groups.

Dimensions of FACT-G	F Values	Level of significance
FACT-G Total	2.17	.073
Physical Well-being	15.216	.000
Social & Family Well-being	1.771	.135
Emotional Well-being	3.787	.05
Functional Well-being	22.038	.000

Therefore, to understand the specific differences in various groups of cancer, Post Hoc DRT was applied. FACT-G Total F value is insignificant. Also the total score is not taken up in this scale as the scoring of sub scale is in reverse order. So no DRT was employed on FACT-G Total. Other values have been shown in the table 5.7.

As indicated in table 5.7 the mean value of control group in **physical well-being** is 3.62 which is lower than all groups of cancer patients. Higher mean scores indicate poor wellbeing. Thus the physical wellbeing was found to be significantly lower in cancer patients of all types taken in the study.

The summary of DRT in table 5.7 further indicates very clearly that, the physical well-being was found to be least affected in the breast cancer group. The cervix cancer group and prostate cancer group did not differ significantly from each other indicating that these two groups were equally worse on physical well-being, and these two were also significantly higher from breast cancer on mean (Poorer QOL). Thus, the reduction in physical well-being of breast cancer patients was much lesser than cervix cancer and prostate cancer patients. However, as already mentioned it did not differ significantly from the lung cancer patients, while lung cancer patients did not differ significantly from cervix and prostate cancer too. In other words like QOL, physical well-being amongst breast cancer patients was also significantly less hit than other types on physical well-being.

Table 5.7: Showing the means and summaries of DRTs applied to the means of various dimensions of well-being of all cancer groups and control group.

Groups & Mean / Dimensions	Control Group	Breast Cancer	Lungs Cancer	Cervix Cancer	Prostate Cancer
Physical well-being	3.62	8.22	9.92	11.62	11.78
Social & family well being	**Control group**	**Cervix cancer**	**Breast cancer**	**Prostate cancer**	**Lung cancer**
	16.66	16.9	17.6	17.68	18.76
Emotional Well-Being	**Lung Cancer**	**Breast Cancer**	**Control group**	**Cervix Cancer**	**Prostate Cancer**
	5.04	5.9	6.16	7.78	7.72
Functional Well-Being	**Cervix Cancer**	**Prostate Cancer**	**Lung Cancer**	**Breast Cancer**	**Control group**
	12.14	13.76	13.88	14.56	20.56

Social & family well-being is a measure ofoffering and getting the required healthy support from family members, friends, and othersignificant associates. The F value for FACT-G Social & family well-being was found to be insignificant, yet DRT was employed. Though the means of all cancer groups are higher but there was no significant difference found between the means of control group, breast, cervix, and prostate cancer groups. Also no significant difference was found between cervix, breast, prostate and lung cancer groups. This indicates that amongst these three groups of cancer patients there was no deterioration in social & family welfare in spite of serious suffering from an acute disease. There is an exception i.e. lung cancer. Patients of lung cancer have shown significantly higher score on social & family well-being. The results **of emotional well-being** indicate that apparently the mean value on emotional well-being of control group was high from lung cancer and breast cancer and these were lower than cervix cancer and prostate cancer. The scoring on this scale is in reverse order. The higher score indicates lower emotional well-being. So lung & breast cancer patients were less poor on emotional well-being. However, none of the cancer groups differed significantly from the control group on emotional well-being, indicating that, cancer did not change the emotional well- being of patients. Further, the means of emotional well-being of cervix cancerand prostate cancer are significantly higher than both the lung cancer and breast cancer patients. It means that the emotional well-being of cervix cancer and prostate cancer patients was poor than lung cancer and breast cancer patients. Thus cancer poses a serious threat to the patients of cervix cancer and prostate cancer. As discussed earlier, better chances of survival in breast cancer could be a cause of lesser worsening in these patients.

Regarding **functional well-being,** as indicated in table 5.7, the mean value of control group is 20.56, which is higher than all groups of cancer patients. Higher mean scores indicate good wellbeing. Thus the functional wellbeing was found to be lower in cancer patients.

The summary of DRT in the above table 5.7 indicates very clearly that the mean value of control group on functional well-being was significantly higher than all other groups, and none of the cancer patients group differed significantly from each other except breast and cervix cancer. In other words the functional well-being was found to be equally worse in each of three groups i.e. the cervix cancer, lung cancer, and prostate cancer group but the cervix cancer group was significantly poor than breast cancer group on functional well-being. In other words the cervix cancer patients have been facing difficulty in carrying out the usual daily routine activity.

Thus cancer in this study has led to poor well- being and the first hypothesis has proved regarding health related well- being also. The cancer patients were significantly lower on FACT-G, though the well-being of different types of cancer patients differed. Breast cancer patients were relatively better than cervix cancer & prostate cancer on physical well-being, than the cervix cancer patients on social & family well-being; than cervix cancer & prostate cancer on emotional well-being; and than the cervix cancer on functional well-being. At the same time cervix cancer was worst on functional well-being and lung cancer was significantly higher on social & family well-being.

The better position of breast cancer patients is understandable in light of fact that the breast cancer is usually easily curable and prognosis is not poor. (http://www.cancer.ca/en/cancer-information/cancer-type/breast/prognosis-and-survival/?region=on, retrieved on 25/8/2018).Recent upgrading/s of thetreatment haveunequivocallyboosted the long term survival of the breast cancer patients at each stage. Breast cancer is the most frequently occurring cancer amongst females with a lifetime risk of up to 12% only and the associated mortality risk is only 5%. This could be a cause of lesser worsening in case of breast cancer (Parkin, Bray, Ferlay, & Pisani, 2005; Peto, Boreham, & Clarke, 2000; Taylor, Davis, & Boyages, 2003). Humpel and Iverson(2007) conducted a study of the well-being by taking 59 prostate cancer and 32 breast cancer survivors. They used the same scale and found a poor well-being on emotional, functional and physical well-being scale of FACT-G. The physical activity played a significant role in helping the patients in recovering from the depression. Most of the patients reported that they were not doing physical activity and they were found to be high on depression. According to Cella (1997), "**FACT-G physical well-being** is the appraisal of lifestyle behavior choices to ensure health, circumvent preventable diseases and conditions and to live in a balanced state of body, mind, and spirit". Somatic health measures reflect on **Physical well-being,** which Cella describes as "Correlates of strength and liveliness, feeling very fit and energetic".

Regarding lung cancer patients there is a misconception in India that lung cancer is a contagious disease. However, lung cancer is not contagious. A tremendous amount of work was performed searching for a contagious cause, but nothing was found which could be confirmed (Epstein, 2001; Shimkin, 1977). But it is sometimes accompanied by tuberculosis. The incidence of pulmonary tuberculosis and lung cancer has been reported to be both simultaneous and sequential in the same patient on the bases of multiple case series and case-control studies (Brenner, Wang, Kleinerman, Wang, Zhang, & Metayer, 2001; Yu, Liao, Hsu, Chen, Liao, & Muo et al., 2011).

The researcher noted that the most of the caretakers think lung cancer to be contagious, though it is not contagious in itself (Welsh, 2011). Many times, the doctors also advise not to go very close to these patients due to other accompanying ailments that could be contagious sometimes. All this should have reduced the social visits of friends & family members but the reverse was found. Here it is important to understand that lung cancer is considered to be more fatal than breast and prostate cancers. The time span of living for patients is relatively short. With this background the higher number of social visits could be owed to the prevalent collectivism in India (Chadda & Deb, 2016). India is well established as a collectivistic nation as compared to many other individualistic cultures like U.S. Over the years, the family culture has slightly changed in India. Though there is deterioration in attachment amongst family members, yet it seems that, in India the family & social system is still well knitted enough and people tend to unite at the time of grief and misery. The care takers are, though under trauma, yet they seem to manage their temper and go to any extent for helping the patient suffering from acute problems. Lung cancer prognosis is generally poor, with the one- and five-year survival rates of 41% and 15%, respectively (The American Cancer Society, 2009). Lung cancer is a fatal than other cancer (Kanwal, Ding, & Cao, 2016). This could be a cause of more visits by people to the lung cancer patients.

Holzner et al., (2004) took the cancer survivors to understand the changes in their SWB by using FACT-G and found that the SWB in different kinds of cancer was different e.g. the breast cancer survivors had shown poor social well-being while the bone marrow transplantation patients had shown lower QOL and the survivors of Hodgkin"s disease were found to be higher on functional and social well-being.

Sexual disfunctioning was found to be very common amongst the cancer patients. It is reported that 42-100% patients start suffering from it after the diagnosis (http://www.cancernetwork.com/article/10165/101698, retrieved on 24/7/18). Donovan et al., (2007) and Jensen et al., (2004) also reported the similar findings. Donovan et al., (2007) found that lesser the interest in sex or more the sexual dysfunction lesser was the satisfaction amongst the women. So this could also be one of the causes to reduce the subjective well-being amongst cervix cancer patients. Higher emotional well-being amongst the lung cancer patients can be understood in cultural context. Frost et al., (2013) conducted a longitudinal study on spiritual well-being and quality of life amongst ovarian cancer patients and their spouses. Though the scale used was different but the SWB was found to be significantly poor. The overall outlook of the patients had changed. The patients felt worried, fatigued and also suffered from insomnia. Emotional well-being is a very important aspect of well-being which usually deteriorates with onset of chronic and acute disease. Emotional wellbeing does not only mean a nonexistence of emotions, but also to the individual capacity to understand the value of one"s emotion and use them in positive direction. An affirmative sense of emotional wellbeing enables an individual to function well in society. Such people are able to easily deal with everyday demands in life. Everyday life emotional well-being also involves identifying, building upon and operating from individual strength.

Hope was the next variable under investigation in the first hypothesis. The score of means have been shown in Table 5.9 and Table 5.8 shows the values of F on hope amongst all the five groups.

Table 5.8: Showing the F values of various dimensions of hope i.e. total score, agency score and pathways score after applying one way ANNOVA.

Variables / Dimensions	F value	Level of significance
Hope (Total)	17.572	.000
Hope (Agency score)	19.848	.000
Hope (Pathways score)	6.920	.000

Table 5.8 indicates that the F values for all the dimensions of Hope i.e. hope (total), agency score and pathways score were found to be significant. Therefore Post Hoc DRT was applied.

Table 5.9 indicates that the mean value of control group in **hope (Total)** being 54.64 is higher than all groups of cancer patients. Higher mean scores indicate better hope. Thus the hope was found to be significantly lower in cancer patients of all types taken in the study.

The summary of DRT in the table 5.9 also indicates very clearly that hope was found to be lowest in cervix cancer group. The mean is significantly lower than lung and breast cancer, but it is not significantly lower from prostate cancer group. Also the difference was found to be insignificant in prostate, lung and breast cancer group. To conclude each type of cancer led to a significant reduction in hope and the cervix cancer patients were affected the most; thus being the worst hit on hope by cancer.

Table 5.9: Showing the means values of various groups and summaries of DRTs applied to the means of various dimensions of hope i.e. total, agency score and pathways score on various cancer groups and control group.

Groups and means / Dimensions of Hope	Cervix cancer	Prostate cancer	Lungs cancer	Breast cancer	Control group
Total score	41.96	44.56	45.6	46.1	54.64
Agency score	**Cervix cancer**	**Prostate cancer**	**Lungs cancer**	**Breast cancer**	**Control groups**
	19.74	20.62	20.88	22.34	28.06
Pathways score	**Cervix cancer**	**Breast Cancer**	**Prostate cancer**	**Lungs Cancer**	**Control group**
	22.22	23.76	23.94	24.72	26.58

As further indicated in the table 5.9, the mean value of control group in **hope agency score** was 28.06 which is higher than all groups of cancer patients. Higher mean scores indicate higher motivation to take the desired pathway. The summary of DRT in the above table 5.9 also indicates very clearly that, the agency score was found to be better in the breast cancer group as it differed significantly from cervix cancer.

However, cervix, prostate and lungs cancer did not differ significantly. As well as there was no significant difference amongst prostate, lung and breast cancer group.

The mean value of control group in **pathways scores** was 26.58 which is significantly higher than all groups of cancer patients. Higher mean scores indicate higher ability to plan pathways. Among the entire four cancer groups lung cancer patients seemed to be least hit but the mean did not differ significantly from the prostate cancer and breast cancer groups. This did differ significantly from cervix cancer group and once again the cervix cancer is the worst hit as this group was significantly lower than breast, prostate and lung cancer patients. No significant difference existed between cervix, breast and prostate cancer groups.

To sum up, hope total, hope agency and pathways had reduced significantly amongst the cancer patients. The first hypothesis pertaining to hope has also proved and cervix cancer patients were found to be the worst hits; differing significantly from breast cancer patients on total and agency score and from lung cancer on pathways score.

In a study of hope by Berendes (2010), hope was found to be inversely related with the symptoms of cancer like pain, fatigue, cough etc. as well as with psychological distress. In another study by Agarwal & Ramakant, (2010), the breast cancer patients were found to have relatively higher hope which was directly proportional to the level of income. Karampour et al., (2018) found moderate levels of hope in the breast cancer patients. In the same way Denewer et al., (2011) found that 34% women suffering from breast cancer had low level of hope, 36.2% had a moderate degree of hope whereas 29.6% person had high level of hope. The results of this study did not show any correlation of hope with socio demographic variables like age, marital status, education and residence. Contradictorily Karampour et al., (2018) and Oztunc et al., (2013) did not find any significant correlation of hope with socio demographic variables. However, anxiety and depression have been found to be correlated with hope Rajandram, (2011), social support Oztunc et al., (2013) and treatment (Oztum et al., 2013; Wakiuchi, 2015). The patients were more optimistic towards the end of the treatment. Regarding social support the higher level of social support was found to be positively correlated with hope.

Hope is also related with anxiety and depression. The oncology patients who have high level of depression and anxiety usually show lower levels of hope. Utne, Miaskowski, Bjordal, Paul, & Rustoen (2010) found in their study conducted on 225 oncology inpatients that the patientswith lower levels of depression and anxiety were higher on hope as compared to the patients with anxiety or depression or both. This is similar to finding of study of 80 oncology in patients in which anxiety and depression were found to be significantly and negatively correlated with hope scores. The findings of Vellone, Rega, Galletti, & Cohen, (2006) were also similar.

In another study Rajandram, Samuel, Samman, Chan, McGrath, & Zwahlen, (2011) found that, hope was negatively correlated with depression ($r = -.55$, $p \leq .001$) and anxiety ($r = -.38$, $p \leq .05$). They and many others have further suggested that hope also plays a role in later adjustment outcome among the patients of cancer. (Chi, 2007; Fadilogli, Cantilav, & Yildirim, 2006; Hammer, Morgenson, & Hall, 2009; Utne, Miaskowski, Bjordal, paul & Rusteon, 2010; Vellone, Rega, Galletti, & Cohen, 2006).

In past studies also there is an evidence of losing hope by the cancer patients (Berendes et al., 2010). Hope is a virtue that provides strength to struggle. As such a method, it has proven helpful in fighting the stress that erupts due to cancer. Hopelessness is the other end of the continuum expected to do the opposite. Loss of hopeheightens the psychologicaldistress and negative thoughts and anticipations about future related negative outcomes. Patients with cancer experience deep hopelessness due to its perception of being fatal with high mortality rate. Hope is serious concern in the cancer patients because once lost the patients will not even struggle to fight with distress at the psychological level. Even the motivation to adhere to the treatment may also reduce. In one of the study (Mcclement & Chochinov, 2008), hope was found to be one of the single key factor that can help the oncology patients with their struggle against the disease, associated uncertainties and distress. Even in the uncertainty of the diagnosis, the capacity to deal with the distress comes through hope.

Agency score tells the motivation to take the pathways to reach the goal thought of achieving. The mean value of agency score in breast cancer patients is significantly higher than cervix cancer and prostate cancer patients. This indicates that, the reduction in motivation of breast cancer was much lesser than cervix cancer and prostate cancer patients. The results in present study clearly indicate that cancer leads to reduction in motivation to reach the goals. Pathways scores reflect upon the ability to plan pathways to desired goals despite obstacles. Thus, the ability to plan for attaining the desired goals was also found to be significantly lower in cancer patients of all types taken in the study.

To summarise, the results of past studies show a mixed trend of hope among the patients of cancer. However, in the present study the score of hope total, agency and pathways score was significantly lower in all types of cancer. Similarly the socio demographic variables as indicated in the past researches do not indicate any kind of a consistent trend in influence the hope. It seems that the disease itself and the association of fatality might be a factor contributing to hope among cancer patients. In the present study all the patients were either of stage 2 or 3 of cancer. This could be a reason for the significantly lower level of hope. It seems necessary to design and apply the hope improving interventions for the patients of cancer. This stands true at least for the Indian population.

Resilience was the fourth and the last variable to be studied while testing the first hypothesis. F value of resilience among five variables has been shown below in table 5.10 .

Table 5.10: Showing the F values of resilience after applying one way ANOVA to the means of various cancer groups and control group.

Variable	F value	Level of significance
Resilience	3.569	.008

Since F value is significant, DRT was employed.

Table 5.11: Showing the means values of various groups and summaries of DRTs applied to the mean resilience scores of various cancer groups and control group.

Groups	Prostate cancer	Cervix cancer	Breast cancer	Lungs cancer	Control group
Mean values	129.38	131.30	140.62	141.92	143.42

It can be seen from table 5.11 that the mean resilience value of control group is 143.42 which is higher than all cancer groups. Higher mean values represent better resilience. *Resilience is one"s ability to recover from hardship or trauma* which is significantly worse than control group in prostate and cervix cancer groups. There exists no significant difference between resilience of prostate and cervix cancer groups, which were lesser on resilience significantly from breast, lung cancer and control group. No significant differences were found among cervix and breast cancer groups; and both of these did not vary significantly from lung cancer group, prostate cancer group and control group. Even there was no significant difference among breast, lung cancer group and control group but these were significantly higher from prostate and cervix cancer group.

Recalling the discussion of quality of life and subjective well-being, prostate cancer and cervix cancer patients were the worst hits. The above results of resilience seem to be in concordance with the earlier findings on quality of life and well-being as the patients of cervix and prostate cancer were significantly lower from the control group on these two variables. Resilience is personality characteristic which allows the strength to fight with stress of various types of in life. Matzka et al.,(2016), found that the cancer patients who had higher level of resilience did not only face the lower psychological distress but were also physically more active. In another study by

Somasundaram and Daevamani (2016), resilience was significantly related to higher level of hope. They also found that social support increases the resilience. Vartak (2015) also found that hope and social support are positively correlated with resilience, emotional adjustment in the patients with the higher level of resilience as well as amongst the normal healthy subjects. Resilience has also been found to be related with lesser level of depression (Kim, Kim& Lee, 2015; Markovitz et al., 2015; Ristevska-Dimitrovska et al., 2015) and anxiety (Giacomo et al., 2016; Markovitz et al., 2015).

Resilience is also important because it can improve the quality of life (Ristevska-Dimitrovska et al., 2015; Ha et al., 2014) and help in alleviation of post-traumatic stress disorder (Ha et al., 2014).

Thus resilience has been shown to be an important indicator of many other factors that play an important role in the disease symptoms and perception in the past studies. One commonality of the same type was found in the present study that cervix and prostate cancer patients were relatively lower on QOL, well-being and also on resilience. Hope was significantly poor in cervix cancer patients. Therefore, it is possible that hope and resilience led to lower QOL and well-being in these patients. It is inferred that hope and resilience play an important role in determining the QOL and well-being amongst the patients of cancer. However, neither studying this is a part of this research nor the time permits to apply the further analysis and verify the same. Major drawback is that the patients taken in each group are not sufficient in number to apply the multiple regression analysis.

To conclude, the first hypothesis seems to have proved as the overall QOL, well-being, hope and resilience were poor in different cancer groups with an exception on dimensions of emotional and social well-being. Social well-being had rather improved though significantly only for lung cancer patients while none of the group deteriorated significantly from control group on emotional well-being. The type of cancer is an important variable to be explored further because the QOL, well-being, hope and resilience had all differed in different types of cancer. Also it is necessary to include the required interventions to raise QOL, subjective well-being, hope and resilience amongst the cancer patients as a part of treatment package. It is important that these interventions need to be designed as per the type of cancer which yet needs to be explored further.

Another goal of the work was to understand how the mental health of cancer patients can be improved. For this as already discussed in chapter 3 while developing the rationale it was decided to study the role of the ways of coping adopted by cancer patients in their mental health. For this, the **second hypothesis** predicted that higher the problem focused coping higher would be the quality of life, subjective well-being, hope and resilience in cancer patients. To test this hypothesis Pearson"s correlation was employed to study the relationship of emotional focused coping & problem focused coping with the total score and dimension, if any, of all the four variables i.e. quality of life, subjective well-being, hope and resilience . The results have been shown below separately for breast, cervix, lung & prostate cancer patients and the control group.

Quality of life and coping

It has been observed in the above discussion pertaining to hypothesis one that cancer is serious threat to the quality of life of the patients suffering from it. Therefore, the correlation of the individual ways adopted for coping with QOL can reflect upon how to improve it. The values of correlations between ways of coping and QOL & its dimensions in all types of cancer groups under taken in the study have been mentioned in table 5.12.

Table 5.12: Showing the correlation between ways of coping and QOL (total and its dimensions) in breast cancer patients.

Ways of coping	Functional scale	Symptom scale	Global health status	Total QOL
Confrontive coping	.039 .393	-.064 .328	.120 .203	.085 .278
Seeking social support	-.040 .391	-.054 .354	-.045 .379	-.117 .209
Planful problem solving	.143 .161	**-.237*** **.049**	.017 .452	-.079 .293
Distancing	-.051 .364	.040 .390	.055 .353	.047 .373
Self- controlling	.162 .130	-.187 .096	.218 .064	.162 .131
Accepting responsibility	-.151 .147	.082 .286	-.023 .437	-.064 .328
Escape-avoidance	-.070 .315	.092 .264	.067 .322	.087 .273
Positive reappraisal	.006 .483	-.061 .336	-.035 .405	-.079 .292
Problem focused coping	.061 .338	-.153 .144	.032 .414	-.056 .350
Emotional focused coping	-.011 .469	-.020 .444	.088 .272	.055 .352

*$P \leq .05$, **$P \leq .01$.

A look on table 5.12 showing the results of breast cancer depicts that neither overall problem focused coping nor overall emotion focused coping was found to be significantly correlated with either the total score of quality of life or any of the dimensions of quality of life i.e. functional scales (Physical, Role, Cognitive, Emotional, and Social Functioning), symptom scales (Fatigue, Pain, and Nausea/Vomiting) and global health status. Regarding various styles of coping, planful problem solving was found to be significantly and negatively correlated with symptom status amongst the breast cancer patients (-.237, $p \leq .049$) indicating that more the planful problem solving lower the score on symptom scale. All other types of coping were not correlated with any of the dimensions of quality of life.

Table 5.13: Showing the correlation between ways of coping and QOL (total and its dimensions) in cervix cancer patients.

Ways of coping	Functional scales	Symptom scales	Global health scales	Total QOL
Confrontive coping	-.040 .392	-.047 .374	.082 .285	-.004 .489
Seeking social support	-.077 .298	.058 .346	**-.351**** **.006**	**-.306*** **.015**
Planful problem solving	.021 .442	-.167 .124	-.143 .161	**-.247*** **.042**
Distancing	.062 .334	-.215 .067	.162 .131	-.001 .497
Self- controlling	-.110 .224	.025 .432	-.179 .107	-.217 .065
Accepting responsibility	.050 .365	-.015 .459	.085 .279	.099 .248
Escape-avoidance	**-.241*** **.046**	.077 .297	-.059 .342	-.178 .108
Positive reappraisal	.091 .266	.025 .432	**-.245*** **.043**	-.110 .223
Problem focused coping	-.043 .384	-.085 .279	-.214 .068	**-.288*** **.021**
Emotional focused coping	-.053 .357	-.026 .428	-.102 .240	-.151 .147

*P≤ .05, **P≤ .01.

In case of cervix cancer it is interesting to note that, both the problem focused coping and emotion focused coping were negatively correlated with total quality of life. However, only problem focused coping was found to be significantly correlated (-.288, P $\leq$ .021); thus proving the reverse of hypothesis. In other words higher the problem focused coping, significantly lower was the total quality of life amongst cervix cancer patients. None of the dimensions of emotion focused coping and problem focused coping were significantly correlated with total quality of life. Regarding the dimensions of QOL, seeking social support was found to be negatively and significantly correlated with global health status and total quality of life (-.351, P $\leq$ .006; -.306, P $\leq$ .015), indicating that more you seek the social support, poorer is the quality of life. This is again in contradiction with the hypothesis. However, while talking to the patients, researcher noted that the patients of cervix cancer in India feel ashamed of showing that they are suffering from cervix cancer as most of these had multiple sexual relationships. So meeting people might have deteriorated their quality of life.

In the same way escape avoidance which is a form of emotional coping (- .241, P $\leq$ .046) was negatively correlated with functional status; planful problem solving was negatively correlated with total quality of life (-.247, P $\leq$ .042); positive reappraisal, again an emotion focused way of coping, was negatively correlated with global health status (- .245, p$\leq$ .043). These results indicated that some of the aspects of emotion focused coping i.e. positive reappraisal and escape avoidance were negatively correlated with some of the dimension of quality of life, In other words higher the emotional coping lower the QOL amongst cervix cancer patients.

Table 5.14: Showing the correlation between ways of coping and QOL (total and its dimensions) in lung cancer patients.

Ways of coping	Functional scales	Symptom scales	Global health status	Total QOL
Confrontive coping	.131 .183	**-.262*** **.033**	.093 .260	-.059 .343
Seeking social support	-.033 .409	.087 .275	.137 .171	.172 .118
Planful problem solving	.063 .332	.020 .446	-.151 .147	-.096 .255
Distancing	.209 .073	-.202 .079	.127 .190	.113 .221
Self- controlling	.233 .052	-.204 .077	.173 .115	.158 .139
Accepting responsibility	**-.265*** **.031**	.174 .113	-.199 .083	**-.263*** **.034**
Escape-avoidance	-.110 .223	.025 .433	-.119 .205	-.205 .079
Positive reappraisal	-.095 .255	-.007 .480	-.195 .087	**-.256*** **.038**
Problem focused coping	.090 .268	-.079 .294	.029 .421	.002 .496
Emotional focused coping	-.004 .490	-.067 .322	-.055 .351	-.126 .194

*P≤ .05, **P≤ .01.

In case of lung cancer the results were found to be similar to breast cancer patients. Neither the problem focused coping nor the emotion focused coping was found to be correlated with either total quality of life or with any of its dimensions. Accepting responsibility was negatively and significantly correlated with functional scale scores (-.265, $P \leq .031$) and with QOL total (-.263, $P \leq .034$). In other words more you accept responsibility more is the deterioration in functioning. Confrontive coping was found to be negatively and significantly correlated with symptom scale (-.262, $P \leq .033$) and positive reappraisal was found to be negatively and significantly correlated with total quality of life (-.256, $P \leq .038$). In other words more the patients make aggressive effort to alter the situation or try the confrontive coping by suggesting some degree of hostility and risk taking, the lesser they suffer from symptoms on cancer; may be because this situation is not possible to alter. Similarly the more one attempts for the positive reappraisal or more one makes efforts to bring or search positivity by focusing on personal growth, poorer will be the quality of life amongst lung cancer patients. It seems that accepting the disease as it is needed for lung cancer patients.

The correlations pertaining to prostate cancer have been shown in table 5.15 on the next page. The table clearly indicates that in prostate cancer, the problem focused coping was significantly and positively correlated with total QOL score (.402, $P \leq .002$) as well as with all of its three dimensions (functional scale: .523, $P \leq .000$; symptom scale: -.402, $P \leq .002$; global health status: .307, $P \leq .004$) indicating that in case of prostate cancer problem focused coping played a significantly positive role in the quality of life including functional status, symptom status and global health status. Negative correlation with symptoms status indicates that higher the Problem Focused coping lower the symptoms, thus better the QOL. On emotion focused coping only functional status was positively and significantly correlated (.309, $P \leq .015$). Thus higher the problem focused coping in all the dimensions higher was the quality of life for the prostate cancer patients. Self-controlling was found to be significantly and positively correlated with functional status (.277, $P \leq .026$) and total quality of life (.281, $P \leq .024$).

Seeking social support seems to have most positive role in maintaining the quality of life as it was found to be highly and positively correlated with total and two of the dimensions i.e. functional status and global health status (total QOL: .401, $P \leq .002$; functional status: .460, $P \leq .000$; global health status: .367, $P \leq .004$). Seeking social support was negatively correlated with symptom status (- .342, $P \leq .008$). This indicates that more you receive the social support lesser the symptoms people may suffer from. Positive reappraisal was positively correlated with total QOL (.333, $P \leq .009$) and with functional scale score (.378, $P \leq .003$).

Table 5.15: Showing the correlation between ways of coping and QOL (total and its dimensions) in prostate cancer patients.

Ways of coping	Functional scales	Symptom scales	Global health scales	TQOL
Confrontive coping	.116 .211	-.067 .321	.016 .456	.045 .377
Seeking social support	**.460**** **.000**	**-.342**** **.008**	**.367**** **.004**	**.401**** **.002**
Planful problem solving	**.520**** **.000**	**-.428**** **.001**	**.388**** **.003**	**.386**** **.003**
Distancing	.160 .134	.020 .445	-.128 .189	.030 .419
Self- controlling	**.277*** **.026**	-.146 .155	.200 .081	**.281*** **.024**
Accepting responsibility	.035 .404	.046 .374	-.123 .198	-.044 .382
Escape-avoidance	.041 .389	-.141 .165	.120 .204	.010 .472
Positive reappraisal	**.378**** **.003**	-.209 .072	.232 .053	**.333**** **.009**
Problem focused coping	**.523**** **.000**	**-.402**** **.002**	**.375**** **.004**	**.402**** **.002**
Emotional focused coping	**.309*** **.015**	-.162 .131	.131 .182	.225 .058

*P≤ .05, **P≤ .01.

On planful problem solving the similar results were observed. Higher was the planful problem solving higher was the total quality of life on functional scales and global health status with a correlation of .386 (P ≤ .003), .520 (P ≤ .000) and .388 (P ≤.003) respectively. Symptom status was again negatively correlated with planful problem solving -.428, (P ≤ .001) showing that higher the planful problem solving lower the symptom status. For prostate cancer patients hypothesis is thus proved and problem focused coping helped these patients to cope in a better way. But some of the emotion focused copings also proved to be good for these patients.

Table 5.16: Showing the correlation between ways of coping and QOL (total andits dimensions) in normal subjects.

Ways of coping	Functional scale	Symptom scale	Global health status	Total QOL
Confrontive coping	-.094 .258	-.083 .283	.058 .344	-.034 .408
Seeking social support	-.115 .213	-.013 .464	.049 .367	-.014 .461
Planful problem solving	-.083 .284	-.052 .359	-.072 .311	-.142 .163
Distancing	-.021 .443	-.025 .432	.085 .280	.061 .336
Self- controlling	.030 .419	-.144 .159	.070 .313	.006 .483
Accepting responsibility	-.082 .285	-.029 .421	**.311* .014**	**.257* .036**
Escape-avoidance	-.147 .154	.134 .176	.226 .057	.230 .054
Positive reappraisal	-.063 .333	-.021 .443	-.082 .287	-.124 .195
Problem focused coping	-.123 .197	-.063 .332	.014 .462	-.081 .288
Emotional focused coping	-.088 .273	-.009 .476	.173 .114	.127 .191

*P≤ .05, **P≤ .01.

The results of normal subjects are quite astonishing because neither problem focused coping nor emotion focused coping were found to be correlated with total quality of life and either of its dimension with an exception of the positive correlation of accepting responsibility with total quality of life (.257, P ≤ .036) and one of its dimensions i.e., global health status (.311, P ≤ .014).

In this way, summarily for the patients of breast cancer, only planful problem solving which is a problem focused coping was significantly and negatively correlated with symptom status, indicating planful problem solving to be good. In cervix cancer patients problem focused coping was correlated with total quality of life but again negatively; indicating problem focused coping to be poor strategy. Escape avoidance and positive reappraisal were also negatively correlated with functional status and symptom status respectively. On the other hand amongst cervix cancer patients problem focused ways of coping i.e., seeking social support and planful problem solving were negatively correlated with global health status and total quality of life respectively.

In lung cancer patients only two ways of coping were correlated with quality of life, i.e. confrontive coping which is a problem focused coping with symptom status and positive reappraisal which is emotion focused coping with total quality of life. Both of these correlations were negative.

In case of prostate cancer the hypothesis had completely proved and the total problem focused coping was found to be positively correlated with the total quality of life as well as all the dimensions. Exactly same was the pattern of significant correlation with planful problem solving. Self-controlling was also found to be positively correlated with functional scales and total quality of life. Interestingly, total emotion focused coping was also positively correlated but with only one dimension i.e. functional scales. Thus regarding QOL for prostate cancer patients the hypothesis has proved. However, in view of the following important highlights the hypothesis for QOL is partially proven. Emotion focused coping dimensions also seem to be good at times for a disease like QOL.

Important highlights

For breast cancer

- For both the breast and cervix cancer patients cancer Problem Focused Coping (PFC) was negatively correlated with QOL which is reverse of the predicted relationship.
- Escape avoidance Emotional Focused Coping (EFC) & planful problem solving (PFC) were negatively correlated with quality of life total for cervix cancer patients.

- For lung cancer patients it was observed that more the confrontive coping lesser the symptoms and more the accepting responsibility poorer the quality of life; thus it seems better to accept the disease „as it is".
- For prostate cancer patients problem focused coping proved highly significant and helped the patients.

Subjective well-being (SWB) and coping

The values of correlations between ways of coping and subjective well-being or health related well-being in all types of cancer groups under taken in the study have been mentioned below in separate tables.

Table 5.17: Showing the correlation between ways of coping and subjective well-being (total& its various dimensions) in the breast cancer patients.

Ways of coping	Physical well-being	Social &family well-being	Emotional well-being	Functional well-being	Total well-being
Confrontive coping	-.073 .306	**.244*** **.044**	.062 .333	**.263*** **.033**	.203 .079
Seeking social support	.026 .429	.230 .054	.033 .410	.136 .174	.193 .090
Planful problem solving	-.149 .151	-.057 .348	-.016 .456	.114 .216	-.082 .287
Distancing	.041 .389	**.294*** **.019**	.190 .094	**.285*** **.022**	**.376**** **.004**
Self- controlling	-.150 .149	.144 .159	.074 .304	**.352**** **.006**	.157 .138
Accepting responsibility	.120 .203	-.196 .086	**.336**** **.009**	.025 .433	.179 .107
Escape-avoidance	.092 .263	.121 .202	.226 .057	.165 .126	**.302*** **.017**
Positive reappraisal	-.039 .394	.122 .200	-.022 .440	.141 .165	.079 .293
Problem focused coping	-.082 .286	.163 .129	.030 .419	.205 .076	.121 .201
Emotional focused coping	.005 .487	.147 .154	.199 .083	**.271*** **.028**	**.289*** **.021**

*P≤ .05, **P≤ .01.

To assess the well-being of cancer patients FACT-G scale was used. It gives a score on physical well-being, social & family well-being, emotional well-being and functional well-being along with total well-being. None of these dimensions were found to be significantly correlated with problem focused coping. With total of emotion focused coping, total well-being (.289, $P \leq .021$) and functional well-being, (.271, $P \leq .028$) were found to be positively and significantly correlated. Regarding the dimensions of problem focused coping, confrontive coping was positively correlated with social & family well-being (.244, $P \leq .044$) and functional well-being (.263, $P \leq .033$). Self-controlling was positively correlated with functional well-being (.352, $P \leq .006$). Regarding emotion focused coping, distancing was found to be positively and significantly correlated with social well-being, functional well-being and total well-being (.294, $P \leq .019$; .285, $P \leq .022$; .376, $P \leq .004$). Accepting responsibility was positively correlated with emotional well-being (.336, $P \leq .009$). Since higher score on emotional well-being indicate poor well-being this means more the accepting responsibility poorer the emotional well-being.

In other words in case of breast cancer patients, emotion focused coping seems to be better overall as it was positively correlated with the total well-being and functional well-being. Accordingly, confrontive coping (PFC) and self-controlling (EFC) & distancing (EFC) seem to be beneficial for improving functional well-being of cancer patients. Similarly seeking social support, confrontive coping and distancing seem to have worked for the breast cancer patients and can be recommended for breast cancer patient. Overall, distancing proved to be most beneficial followed by confrontive coping and then accepting responsibility and self-controlling, which are correlated positively with emotional well-being and functional well-being respectively for the breast cancer patients in this study.

The following section deals with the results of cervix cancer. The results have been depicted in table 5.18 on the next page. The table indicates that for cervix cancer patients none of the ways of coping seem to have worked on overall basis as none were correlated with none of the dimensions of total well-being. Distancing which is an emotional way of coping was negatively and significantly correlated with emotional well-being (-.311, P ≤ .014) and the total well-being (-.256, P ≤ .036). This indicates that the more the distancing or the cognitive effort to detach oneself and minimise the significance of situation, more the emotional well-being and total well-being. Another way of emotion focused coping i.e. escape avoidance had a positive correlation with physical well-being (.277, P ≤ .026) and negative correlation with functional well-being (-.250, P≤.040). In other words more the escape avoidance poorer the physical well-being as well as functional well-being. Regarding the problem focused coping, self-controlling was correlated negatively with social well-being and total well-being (-.282, P ≤ .023; -.256, P ≤ .036).

Table 5.18: Showing the correlation between ways of coping and subjective well-being (total& its various dimensions) in cervix cancer patients.

Ways of coping	Physical well-being	Social &family well-being	Emotional well-being	Functional well-being	Total well-being
Confrontive coping	-.129 .186	-.067 .321	-.223 .060	.108 .227	-.169 .121
Seeking social support	.082 .286	.041 .389	.146 .156	-.172 .116	.049 .367
Planful problem solving	-.105 .234	-.160 .134	**-.272*** **.028**	-.027 .426	**-.294*** **.019**
Distancing	-.226 .057	-.102 .240	**-.311*** **.014**	.183 .101	**-.256*** **.036**
Self- controlling	-.049 .368	**-.282*** **.023**	-.134 .176	-.044 .382	**-.256*** **.036**
Accepting responsibility	.017 .454	.022 .439	.010 .472	.074 .306	.070 .315
Escape-avoidance	**.277*** **.026**	-.226 .057	.131 .183	**-.250*** **.040**	.020 .445
Positive reappraisal	.054 .355	-.048 .370	-.147 .155	-.044 .380	-.073 .307
Problem focused coping	-.075 .303	-.098 .248	-.178 .109	-.051 .362	-.213 .069
Emotional focused coping	.038 .395	-.215 .067	-.149 .152	-.045 .377	-.165 .126

*P≤ .05, **P≤ .01.

Thus self-controlling also influences the well-being in negative way. In the same way planful problem solving also was negatively and significantly correlated to emotional well-being (-.272, $P \leq .028$) and total well-being (-.294, $P \leq .019$) indicating that more the planful problem solving more the emotional well-being for cervix cancer patients. All this is indicating that problem focused coping is not correlated positively with subjective well-being as predicted. Rather it seems to be a poor strategy for well-being amongst breast cancer patients.

Table 5.19: showing the correlation between ways of coping and subjective well-being (total& its various dimensions) in lung cancer patients.

Ways of coping	Physical well-being	Social &family well-being	Emotional well-being	Functional well-being	Total well-being
Confrontive coping	-.205 .077	.050 .366	-.171 .117	**.338**** **.008**	.006 .484
Seeking social support	-.031 .416	.139 .167	.046 .376	-.087 .273	.021 .441
Planful problem solving	.103 .239	**-.304*** **.016**	-.103 .238	.003 .492	-.169 .121
Distancing	**-.262*** **.033**	-.115 .213	-.107 .230	**.269*** **.029**	-.170 .118
Self- controlling	-.179 .107	.083 .284	-.157 .138	.203 .078	-.049 .368
Accepting responsibility	**.290*** **.020**	-.113 .217	**.259*** **.035**	-.050 .365	**.325*** **.011**
Escape-avoidance	.205 .077	**-.246*** **.042**	.114 .215	-.040 .391	.071 .312
Positive reappraisal	-.062 .335	.127 .190	.018 .451	-.055 .353	-.008 .479
Problem focused coping	-.060 .339	-.087 .273	-.129 .186	.132 .181	-.090 .267
Emotional focused coping	.012 .466	-.105 .233	.038 .397	.097 .251	.046 .375

*$P \leq .05$, **$P \leq .01$.

For lung cancer patients again neither problem focused coping nor emotion focused coping were found to be significantly correlated with total well-being or any of its dimensions. Accepting responsibility which is an emotion focused way of coping was found to be significantly correlated with total well-being (.325, $p \leq .011$) and two of the dimensions i.e. physical well-being (.290, $p \leq .020$) and emotional well-being (.259, $p \leq .035$) indicating that accepting responsibility had a negative relationship with well-being. Next major effect was of distancing which is again an emotion focused way of coping. Distancing was negatively correlated with physical well-being (-.262, $p \leq .033$), whereas it was positively correlated with functional well-being (.269, $P \leq .029$). In other words more the distancing better the physical, emotional and functional well- being.

Amongst the problem focused ways of coping confrontive coping was positively correlated with functional well-being (.338, $P \leq .008$) and planful problem solving was negatively correlated with social & family well-being (-.304, $P \leq .016$). Regarding emotion focused coping, escape avoidance was significantly and negatively correlated with social & family well-being (-.246, $P \leq .042$). In the lung cancer patients accepting responsibility had maximum and negative relationship with well-being. Beside this, confrontive coping and distancing were positively correlated with functional well-being. The relationship of distancing was positive with physical and emotional well-being too whereas distancing, escape avoidance and planful problem solving were negatively correlated with physical and social well-being respectively.

Table 5.20: Showing the correlation between ways of coping and subjective well-being (total& its various dimensions) in prostate cancer patients.

Ways of coping	Physical well-being	Social &family well-being	Emotional well-being	Functional well-being	Total well-being
Confrontive coping	-.193 .089	-.039 .393	**-.304*** **.016**	.086 .277	**-.285*** **.022**
Seeking social support	.139 .169	-.004 .490	-.009 .475	.065 .326	.120 .203
Planful problem solving	-.144 .159	-.163 .130	-.175 .113	.137 .172	-.211 .071
Distancing	**-.291*** **.020**	.167 .124	**-.331**** **.009**	.109 .225	**-.257*** **.036**
Self- controlling	.084 .281	.116 .211	-.038 .398	.020 .446	.100 .244
Accepting responsibility	-.028 .422	-.157 .138	-.008 .477	.002 .494	-.107 .229
Escape-avoidance	-.021 .442	.018 .450	-.146 .156	-.066 .323	-.132 .180
Positive reappraisal	-.193 .090	.076 .299	-.160 .134	**.279*** **.025**	-.048 .370
Problem focused coping	-.077 .298	-.097 .251	-.205 .077	.132 .181	-.153 .144
Emotional focused coping	-.154 .143	.083 .284	-.224 .059	.134 .177	-.134 .177

*P≤ .05, **P≤ .01.

For the prostate cancer patients also both problem focused coping and emotion focused coping were not found to be correlated with either total or any other dimensions on subjective well-being. The maximum effect of coping was on total in case of distancing which was negatively correlated with physical well-being, emotional well-being and the total well-being (-.291, P ≤ .020; -.331, P ≤ .009, and -.257, P ≤ .036); thus more the distancing better it is. Another way of emotion focused coping i.e. positive reappraisal was found to be positively correlated with functional well-being (.279, P ≤ .025). Besides this, one of the problem focused coping i.e. confrontive coping was also found to be negatively correlated with emotional well-being (-.304, P ≤ .016) and total well-being (-.285, P ≤ .022), meaning that more the confrontive coping more the emotional well-being. In this way in case of prostate cancer maximum correlation was found to be with distancing which was related positively with well-being. Confrontive coping was also positively related with emotional well-being and total well-being. The only positive and significant correlation was found to be between positive reappraisal which is an emotion focused coping and functional well-being.

The next table indicates the correlation of coping ways and well-being amongst normal healthy controls (Table 5.21). For the normal healthy control overall problem focused coping was not significantly correlated with any of the dimension of subjective well-being. However overall emotion focused coping was found to be positively correlated with emotional well-being (.257, P ≤ .036). Regarding the various dimensions of problem focused coping confrontive coping was found to be significantly and positively correlated with total well-being (.256, P ≤ .036) and functional well-being (.238, P ≤ .048). Also planful problem solving was found to be positively correlated with functional well-being (253, P ≤ .038). While in case of dimensions of emotion focused coping total well-being was found to positively correlated with distancing (.395, P ≤ .002) and positive reappraisal (.295, P ≤ .019). Social and family well-being was positively correlated to distancing (.303, P ≤ .016), positive reappraisal (.304, P ≤ .016) and negatively correlated with escape avoidance (-.257, P ≤ .036). Also escape avoidance was positively correlated with emotional well-being (.258, P ≤ .035).

Table 5.21: Showing the correlation between ways of coping and subjective well-being (total& its various dimensions) in normal subject.

Ways of coping	Physical well-being	Social &family well-being	Emotional well-being	Functional well-being	Total well-being
Confrontive coping	.028 .424	.150 .150	.070 .314	**.238*** **.048**	**.256*** **.036**
Seeking social support	-.039 .395	.007 .480	.018 .451	-.006 .484	-.007 .482
Planful problem solving	-.205 .076	.123 .197	.118 .208	**.253*** **.038**	.172 .116
Distancing	.056 .350	**.303*** **.016**	.147 .154	.234 .051	**.395**** **.002**
Self- controlling	-.037 .399	.101 .243	.191 .092	.119 .205	.193 .089
Accepting responsibility	.020 .445	-.040 .391	.216 .066	.011 .470	.087 .275
Escape-avoidance	.030 .418	**-.257*** **.036**	**.258*** **.035**	-.098 .249	-.078 .294
Positive reappraisal	-.055 .352	**.304*** **.016**	.072 .310	.196 .086	**.295*** **.019**
Problem focused coping	-.093 .260	.119 .205	.088 .272	.207 .075	.179 .107
Emotional focused coping	.005 .486	.088 .272	**.257*** **.036**	.116 .212	.231 .053

*P≤ .05, **P≤ .01.

To summarise the results of correlation of ways of coping with subjective well-being the overall score of emotion focused coping and problem focused coping were not correlated significantly with any of the dimensions except for the emotion focused coping with functional well-being and total well-being in case of breast cancer. This correlation was positive and significant. Another major effect was found to be of distancing which was positively correlated with social well-being, functional well-being and total well-being amongst the breast cancer patients, and with functional well-being for lung cancer patients. This was also positively correlated with social well-being, functional well-being and total well-being for the normal subjects. Further it was negatively correlated with emotional well-being and total well-being amongst cervix cancer patients, with physical well-being and lung cancer patients and with physical well-being, emotional well-being and total well-being amongst the prostate cancer patients.

Important highlights

- Thus different dimensions of both the emotion focused (self-controlling and distancing) and problem focused coping (confrontive coping) were found to be good for health related well-being of **breast cancer** patients. *Distancing was the best* for well-being of breast cancer patients as it improved functional and social well-being.
- For cervix cancer patients distancing and escape avoidance proved to be good ways of coping for emotional well-being and planful problem solving was good for physical well-being.
- For lung cancer patients distancing and escape avoidance ways of emotional focused coping proved better whereas accepting responsibility proved to be a poor strategy.
- For prostate cancer patients again distancing proved to be a good way of coping for physical and emotional well-being. Functional well-being was positively correlated with total and emotional well-being. Problem focused coping was also negatively correlated with social and total well-being.

Hope and coping

The next variable for assessing the correlation with ways of coping was hope. The score on hope was available in three categories, that is, the total score of hope and its two dimensions i.e. agency score and pathways score. The obtained correlations have been depicted in table 5.22 on the following page.

In the patients of breast cancer (Table 5.22) overall problem focused coping was found to correlate positively with total hope score (.299, $P \leq .017$) and the pathway score (.379, .003), whereas overall emotion focused coping was positively correlated with total hope (.316, $P \leq .013$) as well as with both of its dimensions i.e.´pathways score (.278, P ≤ .025) and agency score (.242, P ≤ .045). In other words both of the coping ways were significantly & positively correlated with hope.

Table 5.22: Showing the correlation between ways of coping and hope & its dimensions, i.e. agency score, pathways score and total score in breast cancer patients.

Ways of coping	Agency score	Pathways score	Total hope
Confrontive coping	.149 .151	**.279*** **.025**	**.257*** **.036**
Seeking social support	.046 .376	**.307*** **.015**	.207 .074
Planful problem solving	.113 .217	**.321*** **.011**	**.258*** **.035**
Distancing	.234 .051	**.294*** **.019**	**.319*** **.012**
Self- controlling	**.328**** **.010**	.135 .175	**.287*** **.022**
Accepting responsibility	.063 .332	.160 .133	.133 .178
Escape-avoidance	.131 .183	.210 .071	.205 .076
Positive reappraisal	.117 .209	**.269*** **.029**	.231 .053
Problem focused coping	.124 .195	**.379**** **.003**	**.299*** **.017**
Emotional focused coping	**.242*** **.045**	**.278*** **.025**	**.316*** **.013**

*P≤ .05, **P≤ .01.

Regarding its various dimensions no much correlations were found to be significant. Amongst the problem focused ways of coping, confrontive coping was positively correlated with total hope (.257, P ≤ .036) and pathways score (.279, P ≤ .025). Self-controlling was also found to be correlated with total hope (.287, P ≤ .022) and with agency score (.328, P ≤ .010). Planful problem solving was positively correlated with hope (.258; P ≤ .035) and pathways score (.321, P ≤ .011) indicating planful problem solving to be a positive way of coping for such patients. Distancing was found to be another positive way of coping with reference to hope as the correlation between two was significant and positive (.391; P ≤ .012). Regarding the emotion focused ways of coping, correlation was observed between distancing and pathways score which was .294, (P ≤ .019) and between distancing and Total hope (.319; P≤ .012). Seeking social support was another way of coping that was positively correlated with pathways score of hope(.307, P≤.015).Also positive reappraisal was found to be significantly and positively correlated with pathways score (.269, P ≤ .029).

Table 5.23: Showing the correlation between ways of coping and hope & its dimensions, i.e. agency score, pathways score and total score in cervix cancer patients.

Ways of coping	Agency score	Pathways score	Total hope
Confrontive coping	.150 .148	.070 .314	.133 .179
Seeking social support	-.170 .119	.020 .444	-.097 .250
Planful problem solving	.009 .476	-.006 .484	.002 .494
Distancing	**.242*** **.045**	-.073 .308	.116 .211
Self- controlling	.084 .281	.036 .402	.073 .308
Accepting responsibility	.054 .354	.150 .149	.113 .217
Escape-avoidance	**-.271*** **.028**	-.122 .199	**-.237*** **.049**
Positive reappraisal	-.019 .447	-.022 .440	-.024 .435
Problem focused coping	-.012 .467	.037 .399	.012 .468
Emotional focused coping	.010 .472	-.029 .421	-.009 .476

*P≤ .05, **P≤ .01.

In case of cervix cancer, (Table 5.23) neither problem focused coping nor emotion focused coping was found to be correlated with either the total hope or its dimensions. Regarding various ways of coping only significant correlation was found with escape avoidance, an emotion focused way of coping. With total hope it was negative (-.237, P ≤ .049) and with the agency score also it was negative (-.271, P ≤ .028). Both of these correlations were negative indicating emotion focused ways to be negative ways of coping for these patients. Another way of emotion focused coping, that is, distancing was positively correlated with agency score (.242, P ≤ .045), indicating that distancing can help in focusing on hope agency.

Table 5.24: Showing the correlation between ways of coping and hope & its dimensions, i.e. agency score, pathways score and total score in lung cancer patients.

Ways of coping	Agency score	Pathways score	Total hope
Confrontive coping	**.241*** **.046**	**.351**** **.006**	**.312*** **.014**
Seeking social support	-.159 .135	**-.253*** **.038**	-.215 .067
Planful problem solving	-.037 .398	.063 .333	.000 .499
Distancing	.220 .062	.074 .305	.183 .101
Self –controlling	**.237*** **.049**	**.422**** **.001**	**.338**** **.008**
Accepting responsibility	-.173 .115	-.123 .197	-.171 .118
Escape avoidance	-.068 .319	.011 .470	-.043 .384
Positive reappraisal	-.112 .219	.134 .178	-.023 .437
Problem focused coping	.018 .451	.087 .274	.048 .370
Emotional focused coping	.037 .400	.153 .145	.089 .270

*P≤ .05, **P≤ .01.

For the patients of lung cancer (Table 5.24) again the overall problem focused coping and emotion focused coping did not correlate with hope total as well as its dimensions. Confrontive coping and self-controlling were both positively correlated with total hope (.312, P ≤ .014) and (.338, P ≤ .008), pathway score (.351, P ≤ .006) and (.422, P≤.001) as well as with agency score (.241, P ≤ .046) and (.237, P ≤ .049). One more significant correlation was obtained between seeking social support and pathways score (-.253, P ≤ .038). So for lung cancer patients two of the problem focused ways were correlated as expected in the hypothesis.

Table 5.25: Showing the correlation between ways of coping and hope & its dimensions, i.e. agency score, pathways score and total hope score in prostate cancer patients.

Ways of coping	Agency score	Pathways score	Total hope
Confrontive coping	**.365**** **.005**	.194 .089	**.357**** **.005**
Seeking social support	-.037 .399	.060 .338	.007 .481
Planful problem solving	.220 .062	**.253*** **.038**	**.289*** **.021**
Distancing	**.341**** **.008**	.233 .052	**.362**** **.005**
Self- controlling	.202 .080	.118 .208	.203 .079
Accepting responsibility	-.093 .260	.020 .445	-.054 .356
Escape-avoidance	.018 .451	.074 .305	.052 .360
Positive reappraisal	.073 .308	.146 .157	.129 .186
Problem focused coping	.227 .056	.227 .056	**.280*** **.024**
Emotional focused coping	.170 .119	.192 .091	.221 .061

*P≤ .05, **P≤ .01.

Lastly for prostate cancer patients (Table 5.25) again no correlation were observed with emotion focused coping and problem focused coping except for a positive correlation between problem focused coping and hope (.280, P ≤ .024) indicating that problem focused coping positively correlated with total hope; though none of the dimensions of hope were correlated significantly. One of the problem focused coping and one of the emotion focused coping i.e. confrontive coping and distancing were correlated to hope in a similar way with total hope (.357, P ≤ .005) and (.362, P ≤ .005) respectively as well as with agency score (.365, P ≤ .005) and (.341, P ≤ .008). Another problem focused way of coping i.e. planful problem solving was also positively correlated with total hope (.289, P ≤ .021) and with pathways score (.253, P≤ .038).

Table 5.26: Showing the correlation between ways of coping and hope & its dimensions, i.e. agency score, pathways score and total score in control group.

Ways of coping	Agency score	Pathways score	Total hope
Confrontive coping	.176 .111	.030 .419	.108 .229
Seeking social support	-.094 .258	.058 .344	-.002 .495
Planful problem solving	.185 .099	.038 .397	.118 .207
Distancing	**.328*** **.010**	.176 .111	**.292*** **.020**
Self- controlling	**.318*** **.012**	**.380**** **.003**	**.442**** **.001**
Accepting responsibility	-.025 .432	**.317*** **.013**	.228 .056
Escape-avoidance	**.303*** **.016**	**.237*** **.049**	**.326*** **.010**
Positive reappraisal	.103 .237	.129 .186	.148 .152
Problem focused coping	**.342**** **.008**	.188 .096	**.308*** **.015**
Emotional focused coping	.115 .212	**.264*** **.032**	**.256*** **.037**

*P≤ .05, **P≤ .01.

Regarding the score of normal subjects both the overall problem focused coping and emotion focused coping were found to be positively correlated with total hope (.308, P ≤ .015; .256, P ≤ .037) respectively. Problem focused coping was also positively and significantly correlated with agency score (.342, P ≤ .008). Whereas overall emotion focused coping is positively correlated with pathways score (.264, P ≤ .032). Regarding various dimensions none of the ways of problem focused coping were related significantly with hope and its dimensions. Self-Controlling (.442, $P \leq .001$; .318, $P \leq .012$; .380, $P \leq .003$) and escape avoidance (.326, $P \leq .010$; .303, $P \leq .016$; .237, $P \leq .049$) were positively and significantly correlated with total hope agency and pathway score. Distancing was positively and significantly correlated with total hope (.292, $P \leq .020$) and agency score (.328, $P \leq .010$). Accepting responsibility was found to be significantly correlated with only pathway score (.317, $P \leq .013$).

To summarize these results no consistent trends were found in the correlation of ways of coping with hope amongst various types of cancer. However, overall problem focused coping was positively correlated with total hope in breast cancer patients, prostate cancer patients and healthy control. On the other hand overall emotion focused coping was found to be positively correlated with total hope in breast cancer patients and the normal healthy controls.

Important highlights

- Both problem focused coping and emotional focused coping proved to be good for breast cancer patients. Distancing was better.
- Neither emotion focused coping nor problem focused coping were significantly correlated with hope total of cervix cancer patients. Distancing was positively correlated with agency whereas escape avoidance was negatively correlated with total hope and agency.
- Confrontive coping and self-control as emotion focused coping proved to be good for the lung cancer patients.
- For prostate cancer patients problem focused coping was good, especially planful problem solving.

Resilience and coping

The last variable in the second hypothesis was resilience. The obtained results have been depicted in table 5.27 on the following page. Table evinces that the problem focused coping was found to be positively correlated with resilience in the breast cancer patients (.459, $P \leq .000$), cervix cancer patients (.237, $P \leq .049$), and lung cancer patients (.307, $P \leq .015$). In the prostate cancer and normal subject no such correlation was observed. On the other hand emotion focused coping was found to be positively correlated with resilience amongst breast cancer patients (.492, $P \leq .000$), and lung cancer patients (.307, $P \leq .015$). Normals, cervix cancer patients and prostate cancer patients did not show any correlation with resilience. In the breast cancer patients resilience was also positively correlated with confrontive coping (.343, $P \leq .007$), distancing (.434, $P \leq .001$), self-controlling (.518, $P \leq .000$), seeking social support (.294, $P \leq .019$), escape avoidance (.373, $P \leq .004$), planful problem solving (.460, $P \leq .000$), positive reappraisal (.302, $P \leq .016$). In cervix cancer patient only planful problem solving was positively correlated with resilience (.311, $P \leq .014$) and distancing was also positively correlated (.237, $P \leq .049$).

Table 5.27: Showing the correlation between ways of coping and resilience in breast, cervix, lung & prostate cancer groups and control group.

Ways of coping	Breast cancer	Cervix cancer	Lung cancer	Prostate cancer	Control group
Confrontive coping	**.343**** **.007**	.060 .340	**.495**** **.000**	.190 .093	.081 .287
Seeking social support	**.294*** **.019**	.079 .293	-.047 .374	-.106 .231	.139 .167
Planful problem solving	**.460**** **.000**	**.311*** **.014**	.117 .209	**.370**** **.004**	.095 .255
Distancing	**.434**** **.001**	**.237*** **.049**	**.286*** **.022**	.078 .294	.210 .072
Self- controlling	**.518**** **.000**	.049 .368	**.523**** **.000**	.223 .060	.111 .221
Accepting responsibility	.176 .111	.014 .461	-.054 .356	-.195 .088	.129 .186
Escape-avoidance	**.373**** **.004**	-.042 .387	.130 .183	-.119 .205	.004 .488
Positive reappraisal	**.302*** **.016**	.163 .128	.121 .201	.092 .262	.186 .098
Problem focused coping	**.459**** **.000**	**.237*** **.049**	**.307*** **.015**	.203 .079	.133 .178
Emotional focused coping	**.492**** **.000**	.143 .160	**.307*** **.015**	.040 .390	.169 .121

*$P \leq .05$, **$P \leq .01$.

In lung cancer patients confrontive coping, distancing and self-controlling were positively correlated with resilience with a correlation coefficient of .495, ($p \leq -.000$), .286, ($p \leq .022$) and .523, ($p \leq .000$) respectively. In prostate cancer patients none of the ways of coping except planful problem solving was found to be significant. The positive correlation between resilience and planful problem solving was .370 which is significant at .004 levels. In the normal subjects there were no any positive correlations observed between the ways of coping and resilience.

A look at the table 5.27 showing the results of normal healthy control depicts that neither overall problem focused coping nor overall emotion focused coping was found to be significantly correlated with resilience. Regarding various dimensions of problem focused coping and emotion focused coping none of them were significantly correlated with resilience.

Important highlights

- For breast cancer patients both problem focused coping and emotion focused coping were positively correlated with resilience, except for dimension accepting responsibility which is emotion focused coping.
- For cervix cancer patients problem focused coping total and one of its dimension i.e. planful problem solving were correlated positively with resilience. While only one type of emotional coping i.e. distancing was also positively correlated.
- For lung cancer patients, both problem focused coping and emotion focused coping in total were positively correlated and two ways of problem focused coping (Confrontive coping and Self controlling) as well as only one way of emotion focused coping (Distancing) were positively correlated with resilience.
- For prostate cancer patients ways of coping do not seem to help in developing resilience as only planful problem solving way of problem focused coping was positively correlated.

The related past studies also indicate different kinds of trends (Reynolds et al., 2000). Amongst the breast cancer survivors for both black and white women, emotion focused coping, particularly "the expression of emotions" was more positively correlated with survival. Similarly in another study by (Yahaya et al., 2015) also, the use of emotion focused coping was found to be positively correlated with physical and psychological distress. Social support seeking strategy followed by problem solving and avoiding strategies were found to be the most beneficial way of coping amongst cancer patients (Karabulutlu et al., 2010). Seeking social support followed by planful problem solving and distancing were found to be most frequently used by breast cancer patients by Subhashini (2011). In another study, that was conducted by Deng et al., (2017), problem focused coping styles were found to have a direct relationship with quality of life in breast cancer patients. From the early studies also it seems that there exist no consistent trend on the relationship of total problem focused coping and emotion focused coping, though overall emotion focused coping seems to be better in more studies for dealing with the disease oriented stress, anxiety or depression. For cancer as discussed above, seeking social support seems to be the best way of coping that can improve the quality of life followed by planful problem solving and distancing or avoiding. However, no such relationship was observed consistently in the present study, though seeking social support proved to be good for some dimensions of QOL, well- being and hope. Cervix cancer patients were rather found to be an exception as they confessed that it is shameful and they rather felt embarrassed while meeting friends. As already mentioned most of the patients had multiple sex partners and owed their problem of cancer to this practice.

In one study by Zhang, Gao, Wang, & Wu, (2010) hope was found to be negatively correlated with emotion focused coping amongst breast cancer patients. Karampour, Malek, Fereidooni-Moghadam, Zarea, & Masoudi, (2018) found in their study that there was a linear but reverse relationship between hopelessness and social support. Confrontive coping had a significant correlation with hope of breast cancer, lung cancer and prostate cancer patients. Self-controlling also had a significant correlation in breast cancer and lung cancer patients. No any other consistent trends were observed.

In one of the studies resilience was found to be associated with lower hopelessness and high perceived social support (Oztunc, Yesil, Paydas, & Erdogan, 2013). Resilience was found to be positively correlated with hope and family support amongst breast cancer patients (Kim, Kim,& Lee, 2015) and cancer patients (Vartak, 2015). Resilience was also found to be positively correlated with family support (Kim, Kim,& Lee, 2015; Oztunc, Yesil, Paydas, & Erdogan, 2013; Somasunderam & Daevamani, 2016; & Vartak, 2015).

In a study conducted by Ransom, Jacobson, Schmidt, & Andrykowski (2005), it was found that the early breast cancer patients over concentrated on their symptoms. However, this over concentration is a poor and maladaptive strategy whereas information seeking yielded much beneficial effects for the physical recovery of the patients. In a study by Maleknia & Kahrazei (2015) QOL was found to be related with both i.e., emotion focused and problem focused strategies. Two dimensions that is total quality score and the functional symptoms score were found to be positively correlated with problem focused coping and negatively correlated with emotion focused coping. This is suggested that problem focused coping was a better strategy to cope with cancer.

However, it is unfortunate that most of the patients use emotion focused coping more frequently than the problem focused coping (Ahadi et al, 2014; Kim et al. 2003; Yahaya et al. 2015). At the same time, there are evidences indicating the adoption of mixed styles of coping or using some dimensions of problem focused and emotion focused styles simultaneously (Ahadi et al., 2014; Reynolds et al., 2000). In the present piece of work also somewhat mixed patterns were observed as indicated in table 5.28 given at the end of discussion.

Ahadi, Delaver, & Rostami, (2014) found that most of the cancer patients used emotion focused coping strategy more than the healthy patients. They frequently used confrontive coping, escape avoidance and social support. Self- controlling, accepting responsibility, Plan full problem solving and positive appraisal were hardly ever used by these patients. The patients of ovarian cancer were found to use acceptance, emotional support and religion as the problem focused coping strategies whereas self-destruction, venting and behavioral disengagement were used quite frequently as emotion focused strategies by these patients. In this study quality of life was found to be positively correlated with problem focused coping in comparison to emotion focused coping. Interestingly in another study the quality of life was found to be positively correlated with avoidant coping style indicating that emotion focused coping is better for these patients. In this study the patients were advised to use emotion focused coping strategies (Jalal et al., 2015).

In the same way, in a study by Ptacek, Gregory, Piece, Ptacek, & Cheryl Nogel, (1999), it was found that the emotion focused strategies were related with the current adjustment. This again indicates the emotion focused strategies to be better. In a study by Nunes, Melo, Junior, & Eulalio, (2016) it was found that the problem focused strategy was able to explain the patient in a better way indicating that focus on the problem helps in the improvement of well- being and adaptation towards the health indicating that the ways of coping were significantly related with anxiety. There was a positive significant association between the trait anxiety and the problem focused strategies.

In another study by Oancea, Suciu, Timar, Papavo, Raica, & Burlacu, (2018) again the anxiety scores were significantly and positively correlated with the social support and avoidance coping style. This indicates that more the avoidance and more the social support lower was the anxiety. Hu, Xiao, Peng, Kuang, & He, (2018) observed that higher levels of resilience and social support help in lowering the levels of anxiety and depression among the patients of cancer.

To conclude it is difficult to say that which of the coping strategies are better to deal with cancer because the studies are contradictory and some of the studies show emotion focused coping to be better whereas other studies show problem focused coping to be better. The results are not consistent and nothing much can be concluded. May be the individual differences and other personality factors as well as the environmental factors are important interacting factors here. There can be some mediating or moderating effects of such factors. However, it is clear that various indicators of mental health are differently correlated and separate ways may be required for each individual to enhance different indicators of positive mental health.

It is interesting to note that for the other diseases also the results are usually not very consistent. However, in case of cancer distancing has been found and recommended to be one of the good strategies. The more you stop discussing and focusing upon the symptoms better is the quality of life and the subjective well-being of the cancer patients. In the present study also distancing was found to be positively correlated with agency score & total hope (dimension of hope) in prostate cancer, functional well-being (Dimension of subjective well-being) and resilience in lung cancer group, agency score (Dimension of hope) and resilience in cervix cancer patients and in breast cancer patients social and family well-being, functional well-being & total well-being (Dimension of subjective well-being), resilience and pathways score and total hope (Dimensions of hope).

Although the hypothesis that, higher the problem focused coping higher the quality of life well-being, hope and resilience has not proved yet these results are similar to the conclusion drawn by Lazarus and Folkman (1984) and Mccrae (1984). The situational correlates have been shown to be determinants of ways of coping adopted by individuals. The use of problem focused coping was found to be more in the situations appraised as challengeable whereas emotion focused coping is expected to be more in the situation perceived to be changeable by the individual. Also problem focused coping was found to be more prevalent in the work related situation and emotion focused coping was found to be adapted more while dealing with the family and health situation. Cancer is often perceived to be a non-transitional situation due to the fatality associated with it. This way the results seem to be in congruence with the conclusion drawn by Lazarus and Folkman. Similarly though there are no studies available on hope but it was highlighted in the last section that the hope reduced amongst the cancer patients, as found in the present study. Regarding the other illnesses or diseases hope has been found to be an important positive indicator as has been discussed in the last section for cancer also.

It is recommended on the basis of this study and discussion that distancing, social support are some of the beautiful strategies which help the patients in forgetting the symptoms and raise the hope. Therefore, the caretakers and the patients must focus on the family support and the other social support that can be received and given to these patients.

After deliberating so much on ways of coping it seems highly meaningful to analyse the pattern of frequency of ways of coping adopted by patients in the present study. Though it was not a part of hypothesis, but a count of frequency can guide on the changes that need to be brought in ways of coping. Following is the account of frequency of ways of coping being used by the patients.

For calculating the frequency of the subjects being high or low on using a particular strategy, the means and SD of each group were calculated separately. Those higher than Mean + SD were considered to be high while those lower than Mean- SD were considered to be low on use of that coping style. The frequencies thus obtained have been shown in table 5.28.

The table 5.28 clearly shows that the 38 patients were high on using problem focused coping while 47 patients were low on it; thus problem focused coping was used by lesser number of cancer patients. Similarly number of patients using high emotion focused coping was 43 while 36 were low on it indicating a higher frequency of the patients using emotional focused coping. Frequency of those high on problem focused coping was lower (38) than those high on emotion focused coping (43). In simple words a much higher number of patients were using emotion focused coping in this study. Confrontive coping was the next frequently used way of coping. 48 subjects were high on it while almost an equal number of 47 were low on this. In fact on most of the ways of coping there was no much difference in the frequencies of those high or low on different ways of coping.

Regarding its various dimensions in problem focused way of coping planful problem solving was being used by a higher number of patients i.e. 57 as compared to 47 patients of cancer who were low on it. The results discussed above indicated that using planful problem solving is a positive way of coping for breast cancer patients whereas for cervix cancer patients it did not prove to be very good. Regarding emotion focused coping distancing has been found to be constantly good. Therefore, this is a negative finding that only 31 cancer patients were high on using the distancing as compared to 43 cancer patients who were low on distancing.

Table 5.28: Showing the frequency of ways of coping (problem focused coping and emotion focused coping) used by breast, cervix, lung & prostate cancer patients and control group.

	Breast cancer		Cervix cancer		Lung cancer		Prostate cancer		Control group		Total	
Ways of coping	High	Low	High	Low	High	Low	High	Low	High	Low	High	Low
Confrontive coping	10	12	12	8	6	11	10	8	10	8	48	47
Distancing	7	12	6	9	9	8	4	7	5	7	31	43
Self-controlling	10	7	10	8	10	9	9	11	8	8	47	43
Seeking social support	9	10	11	9	11	7	9	10	6	8	46	44
Accepting responsibility	11	11	10	8	7	8	8	6	9	7	45	40
Escape avoidance	9	6	8	10	11	8	5	8	6	11	39	43
Planful problem solving	15	6	10	8	11	12	13	10	8	11	57	47
Positive reappraisal	8	9	2	9	9	7	10	3	3	4	32	32
Emotional focused coping	11	7	7	6	10	10	9	5	6	8	43	36
Problem focused coping	6	10	5	9	9	7	10	12	8	9	38	47
Total	96	90	81	84	93	87	87	80	69	81		

There is a need to create this awareness amongst the cancer patients that distancing is a positive way of coping with cancer. Another emotion focused way of coping, that is, accepting responsibility was also found to be being using by 45 patients as compared to 40 patients who were poor on it. The results discussed above have indicated that this strategy was found to be poor for functional scale in QOL, physical and emotional well-being of lung cancer, emotional well-being of breast cancer.

However, this is just a picture drawn out of curiosity and guidance. Chi square could be applied to test the significance of differences in these observed differences. But further statistical analysis was not applied because this was not the actual aim of the study.

The **last two hypothesis** of the study pertained to the effect of progressive muscle relaxation on the cancer patients. **Third hypothesis** predicted that progressive muscle relaxation would improve the QOL well-being, (FACT-G), hope and resilience amongst patients of breast, cervix, lung and prostate cancer. The **fourth hypothesis** predicted that the fatigue as well as hospital anxiety & depression would reduce as a result of practicing PMR. To test this, the patients were given progressive muscle relaxation through a CD by Batra (2008) for 15 sessions on alternate days. Now the patients were again assessed. The obtained before and after mean values of all these variables in different types of cancers were now statistically tested by applying t on the pre and post means, as shown in table 5.29 on the next page.

Table 5.29 is showing the pre and post PMR means, t values and the level of significance for the quality of life and its various dimensions for breast, cervix, lung and prostate cancer patients. The table clearly indicates that the QOL for the breast cancer patients on total score of QOL, functional scales, symptom scales and global health status had significantly improved. Similarly the table further indicates that the breast cancer patients, lung cancer patients, the prostate cancer patients and the cervix cancer patients improved on quality of life and all its dimensions in a significant way.This is a very positive finding of this study, indicating that symptoms had reduced, functional status (role & cognitive) had improved and their personal evaluation on global health status had also improved. Thus the total QOL significantly improved in the cancer patients of all types studied here by experiencing PMR for 15 sessions on each alternate day.

Table 5.29: Showing pre and post PMR mean scores of quality of life total and its various dimensions, t values and level of significance for breast, cervix, lung and prostate cancer patients.

Quality of life total	Pre PMR mean	Post PMR mean	t value	Level of significance
Breast cancer	161.59	169.74	4.192	.002
Cervix cancer	144.38	155.84	4.238	.002
Lung cancer	153.03	161.50	2.929	.017
Prostate cancer	157.44	165.67	4.285	.002
Functional scales QOL				
Quality of life Functional status	**Pre PMR mean**	**Post PMR mean**	**t value**	**Level of significance**
Breast cancer	61.33	70.44	4.75	.001
Cervix cancer	47.33	59.111	8.615	.000
Lung cancer	63.71	70.66	3.123	.012
Prostate cancer	65.778	73.555	6.014	.000
Symptom scales QOL				
Quality of life Symptom status	**Pre PMR mean**	**Post PMR mean**	**t value**	**Level of significance**
Breast cancer	40.257	28.461	4.54	.001
Cervix cancer	52.05	39.23	10.112	.000
Lung cancer	38.49	30	5.53	.000
Prostate cancer	36.665	27.949	5.665	.000
Global health status QOL				
Quality of life Global status	**Pre PMR mean**	**Post PMR mean**	**t value**	**Level of significance**
Breast cancer	60.001	70.833	4.994	.001
Cervix cancer	45.001	57.5	6.709	.000
Lung cancer	50.833	60.833	3.087	.013
Prostate cancer	54.999	64.167	4.714	.001

Table 5.30: Showing pre and post PMR mean values, t values and level of significance of well-being and its various dimensions total in breast, cervix, lung and prostate cancer patients.

Physical well-being				
FACT-G Physical well-being	**Pre PMR mean**	**Post PMR mean**	**t value**	**Level of significance**
Breast cancer	12.7	11.7	2.535	.032
Cervix cancer	18.7	17.5	3.087	.013
Lung cancer	12.8	12	2.449	.037
Prostate cancer	13	12	3.873	.004
Social & family well-being				
FACT-G Social and family well-being	**Pre PMR mean**	**Post PMR mean**	**t value**	**Level of significance**
Breast cancer	16.9	18	3.161	.012
Cervix cancer	17.1	18.4	2.751	.022
Lung cancer	15.7	16.9	3.087	.013
Prostate cancer	14.4	16	6	.000
Emotional well-being				
Fact G emotional well-being	**Pre PMR mean**	**Post PMR mean**	**t value**	**Level of significance**
Breast cancer	7.4	6.8	2.714	.024
Cervix cancer	10.5	9.6	3.857	.004
Lung cancer	7.7	7	2.689	.025
Prostate cancer	10.9	9.8	3.498	.007
Functional well-being				
Fact G functional well-being	**Pre PMR mean**	**Post PMR mean**	**t value**	**Level of significance**
Breast cancer	12.1	13.1	3.857	.004
Cervix cancer	8.9	9.9	3.357	.008
Lung cancer	8.4	9.4	4.743	.001
Prostate cancer	12.5	13.4	2.586	.029

Table 5.30 shows the pre post means of physical well-being, social & family well-being, emotional well-being and functional well- being of all the four types of cancer with t values and the level of significance. The pre post means of total well-being were not calculated in the view of reverse scoring. Therefore, the means are not able to show the exact position as they negate the effect of each other. For breast cancer patients all four types of well-being were found to have significantly improved. In cervix cancer patients also all the four types of well-being were found to significantly improve after the progressive muscle relaxation. Exactlysame pattern was observed for the other two types of cancer i.e. prostate and lungs also. This indicates that there was a significant improvement in all the four types of cancer after progressive muscle relaxation on well-being that is the physical, social & family, emotional as well as functional well-being. The hypothesis for well-being has thus proved and PMR has led to an improvement in well-being amongst cancer patients.

Next table 5.31 shows the resilience before and after progressive muscle relaxation practice

Table 5.31: Showing pre and post PMR mean values, t values and level of significance of resilience in breast, cervix, lung and prostate cancer patients.

Resilience	Pre PMR mean	Post PMR mean	t value	Level of significance
Breast cancer	125.4	129.1	3.177	.011
Cervix cancer	120.7	124.1	4.083	.003
Lung cancer	126.5	131.4	2.735	.023
Prostate cancer	121.4	124.4	2.405	.040

Table 5.31 indicates that the resilience had improved and the value was found to be significant at .01 levels. These results are highly positive and supportive results for the cancer patients. In the earlier section it has already been discussed that high resilience is related to lowering of anxiety and depression. Though many authors and researchers have taken resilience to be a trait which is not easy to change. But the resilience has increased significantly by giving the progressive muscle relaxation practice for 30 days on the alternate days, that is, for the 15 sessions only. This proves the hypothesis for resilience also.

Table 5.32 below is showing the values of hope for all types of cancer. The total value of hope and both of its dimensions, that is, the agency score and the pathways score were found to have significantly improved in case of breast cancer patients. These have significantly improved for the cervix cancer, lung cancer as well as for the prostate cancer also as the t values are all significant. The hypothesis for hope has also proved indicating that practicing progressive muscle for 30 days on alternative sessions was able to significantly enhance the hope level in total as well as on both of its dimensions that is the agency and pathways. Again this is also a wonderful finding regarding the effects of progressive muscle relaxation. This technique has been found to increase the hope of the patients of the other diseases as well. Thus the third hypothesis had proved.

Table 5.32 Showing pre and post PMR mean values, t values and level of significance of hope and its various dimensions total in breast, cervix, lung and prostate cancer patients.

Hope total	Pre PMR mean	Post PMR mean	t value	Level of significance
Breast cancer	35.2	38.7	3.452	.007
Cervix cancer	33	35.2	8.82	.000
Lung cancer	32	34.6	6.5	.000
Prostate cancer	35.5	37.4	3.767	.004
Agency score				
Hope agency score	**Pre PMR mean**	**Post PMR mean**	**t value**	**Level of significance**
Breast cancer	14.6	16.3	2.325	.045
Cervix cancer	13.6	15.2	7.236	.000
Lung cancer	11	12.7	6.53	.000
Prostate cancer	13.1	14.4	3.545	.006
Pathways score				
Hope Pathways score	**Pre PMR mean**	**Post PMR mean**	**t value**	**Level of significance**
Breast cancer	20.6	22.4	5.014	.001
Cervix cancer	19.4	20	3.674	.005
Lung cancer	21	21.9	3.857	.004
Prostate cancer	22.4	23	2.714	.024

To verify the last hypothesis the variables studied were fatigue and hospital anxiety & depression amongst the cancer patients which is a very serious issue for these patients, Multi fatigue inventory was used for the purpose which measured general, physical and mental fatigue. The reduced activity and reduced motivation were also studied.

Table 5.33: Showing pre and post PMR mean values, t values and level of significance of fatigue and its various dimensions total in breast, cervix, lung and prostate cancer patients.

Total fatigue	Pre PMR mean	Post PMR mean	t value	Level of significance
Breast cancer	73.1	65.4	3.893	.004
Cervix cancer	79.3	70.8	7.965	.000
Lung cancer	72.3	65.2	5.31	.000
Prostate cancer	63.9	58.7	3.492	.007
General fatigue				
General fatigue	**Pre PMR mean**	**Post PMR mean**	**t value**	**Level of significance**
Breast cancer	15.8	14.3	2.355	.043
Cervix cancer	15.7	14.2	3.737	.005
Lung cancer	15.1	13.3	3.038	.014
Prostate cancer	14.6	12.9	2.486	.035
Physical fatigue				
Physical fatigue	**Pre PMR mean**	**Post PMR mean**	**t value**	**Level of significance**
Breast cancer	18	16.2	5.511	.000
Cervix cancer	17.7	16	4.295	.002
Lung cancer	18.2	16.4	4.323	.002
Prostate cancer	13.4	12.7	2.333	.045
Mental fatigue				
Mental fatigue	**Pre PMR mean**	**Post PMR mean**	**t value**	**Level of significance**
Breast cancer	12.2	11	2.343	.044
Cervix cancer	13.6	12.6	2.372	.042
Lung cancer	11.8	10.8	2.739	.023
Prostate cancer	12.8	11.8	2.372	.042

Reduced activity				
Reduced activity	**Pre PMR mean**	**Post PMR mean**	**t value**	**Level of significance**
Breast cancer	16.4	14.8	2.667	.026
Cervix cancer	19	16	9	.000
Lung cancer	17	15.4	3.073	.013
Prostate cancer	13.5	12.5	3	.015
Reduced motivation				
Reduced motivation	**Pre PMR mean**	**Post PMR mean**	**t value**	**Level of significance**
Breast cancer	10.7	9.1	2.278	.049
Cervix cancer	13.3	12	2.751	.022
Lung cancer	10.2	9.3	2.377	.041
Prostate cancer	9.6	8.8	2.449	.037

A careful look at table number 5.33 clearly indicates that all four types of patients of cancer had significantly improved in all the dimensions taken in the multi fatigue inventory. In other words the general fatigue, mental fatigue, physical fatigue and the total fatigue had significantly improved. However, the reduced activity and reduced motivation were also found to be significantly reduced. In other words, activity level and motivation had improved by PMR practice. This is also a positive finding as the fatigue had improved significantly.

The last variable studied in this hypothesis was Hospital anxiety & depression. The scores and the t values with the level of significance have been shown in table 5.34.

Table 5.34: Showing pre and post PMR mean values, t values and level of significance of hospital anxiety and depression in breast, cervix, lung and prostate cancer patients.

Hospital anxiety and depression total	Pre PMR mean	Post PMR mean	t value	Level of significance
Breast cancer	7.2	4.8	2.714	.024
Cervix cancer	24.8	21.2	3.857	.004
Lung cancer	18.4	15.2	3.207	.011
Prostate cancer	21.6	17.6	6.708	.000
Anxiety				
Anxiety	**Pre PMR mean**	**Post PMR mean**	**t value**	**Level of significance**
Breast cancer	11.6	10	2.449	.037
Cervix cancer	11.2	9.2	3	.015
Lung cancer	5.2	3.6	2.449	.037
Prostate cancer	6.4	4.8	2.449	.037
Depression				
Depression	**Pre PMR mean**	**Post PMR mean**	**t value**	**Level of significance**
Breast cancer	18.8	14.8	3.354	.008
Cervix cancer	13.6	12	2.449	.037
Lung cancer	13.2	11.6	2.449	.037
Prostate cancer	15.2	12.8	3.674	.005

Table 5.34 clearly again indicates that both the anxiety & depression had significantly reduced in all the four types of the patients of cancer. It is concluded that hypotheses 3 and 4 have proved.

The past studies are also indicating the similar findings. In a study by Lerman et al., (1990) it was observed that progressive muscle relaxation reduced the nausea and the vomiting. The same results were found in studies by Molassiotis (2000) and Molassiotis, Yanq, Yam, Chan, & Mok, (2002). Molassiotis et al., (2002) indicated that the chemotherapy induced effects had reduced by PMR and it was suggested that PMR can be called as antiemetic therapy.

The advantage in this therapy is that this is an easy to self-administer therapy. Isa et al., (2013) trained the prostate cancer patients on brief PMR and breathing. When the patients were able to achieve the mastery they were asked to practice PMR daily for 6 months at home. After 6 months, though depression could not improve significantly but a significant reduction was found in anxiety levels. Anxiety and depression in the cancer patients were found to reduce in many studies (Kim & Seo, 2010; Isa et al., 2013; Tsitsi et al., 2017; & Pelekasis et al., (2017). Depression was also found to reduce in many studies Isa et al., 2013; Pathak et al., 2015; & Charalambous et al., 2015). Pelekasis (2016) conducted a systematic review and meta-analysis on eleven articles selected after employing relevant exclusion and inclusion criterion. The obtained results indicated that, PMR had significantly improved the condition of patients by having a significant impact on chemotherapy related complication like nausea and anxiety in eight studies. He suggested that there is a need to conduct further studies on how the health care staff can advise the patients of cancer about such effects of PMR.

Quality of life was also found to be improved in some studies (Molassiotis et al., 2002; Pathak et al., 2013; Yoo et al., 2005). Yoo et al., (2005), had used PMRT and guided imagery (GI). They found that the breast cancer patients not only reported significantly less anticipatory nausea but also the post chemotherapy nausea and vomiting. PMRT and GI led to significantly lower level of anxiety, depression as well as hostility. It also improved the QOL of the hospitalized cancer patients who were receiving radiotherapy in an Indian study by Pathak et al., (2013). Thus there are number of studies indicating an improvement amongst the cancer patients undergoing either chemotherapy or radiotherapy.

The sleep quality and fatigue have also been found to improve (Demiralp et al., 2010). Fatigue in terms of physical symptoms was also found to be reduced in the studies conducted by Gupta et al. (2016) and Shahriari et al. (2017). Hospital stay was also found to reduce in a study by Zhou et al.,(2014).

In the past researches, no studies could be found to compare the effect of PMR on hope and resilience. However, there are evidences indicating the positive impact of

PMR on well-being as measured by FACT G. Parás-Bravoet al., (2017) conducted a study on 272 cancer patients who had different pathology but were showing anxiety symptoms. These patients practiced brief version of PMR for one month. The overall HRQOL on FACT G score along with physical well-being, social & family well-being, emotional well-being and functional well-being were found to significantly improve. They have recommended relaxation technique as complimentary technique for cancer patients. This study has clearly indicated that the results were ditto for all types of cancer. It won't be erroneous to say that PMR should be an integral part of the treatment package for the patients of cancer.

To summarise it can be said that though there are no enough number of studies available that directly pertain to on the variables studied in present research yet there is no doubt that the results of the effect of PMR training have been found to be consistent and these are very positive. Past studies are indicating that PMR can reduce the stress caused by cancer, which is expected to result in improving the quality of life as well as the subjective well-being of the cancer patients. There is no doubt that PMR can help the cancer patients in multiple ways. Raising hope and resilience by PMR is going to prove to be a tool of strength to face the challenge and fight with it. As it is, this kind of the training is much easier than training the patients on different ways of coping to be adopted; the results of which are yet inconsistent and do not seem to give any direction about how to guide the cancer patients. The consistency of the results for different variables obtained in the present study and the results obtained in the past studies have strengthened this confidence further. The technique is very economical which can be imparted through a CD in the Hospital even if there are no trained counselors. The doctors must recommend it to all the patients of cancer, so that they can live a happy life even if it is short for them.

To conclude the results of whole chapter, hypothesis one has proved as in most of the groups of cancer patients QOL, SWB, hope & resilience were found to be lowered. Regarding hypothesis two no any consistent direction in patterns of coping with cancer could be observed and the hypothesis predicting that higher the problem focused coping higher would be the quality of life, subjective well-being, hope and resilience in both the patients and healthy controls did not prove. The last two hypotheses predicted progressive muscle relaxation would enhance the quality of life, subjective well-being, resilience, hope and would reduce the fatigue and hospital anxiety. Both have been proved to conclude that the PMR is a good adjunctive therapy for cancer patients.

Implications

The results of the present study have clearly indicated in the 1st phase that the cancer, be it of any type, brings deterioration in mental health of the patients suffering from it. Positive mental health indicators studied in the present correct piece of research included quality of life, health related well-being, hope and resilience. All the indicators proved to have reduced. This is a serious matter and a strong humane concern, which also reflects upon the strong need and relevance of taking steps to enhance the mental health of each cancer patients as soon as one is diagnosed. It is important to look at the ways of maintaining the quality of life and well-being of the patients. In fact better quality of life, well-being, hope and resilience definitely play a very positive role in maintaining the physical health, as well as the will power to fight with the disease. It is important to maintain the „desire of living" which will further motivate the cancer patient to actively fight the disease. Therefore, researchers, and health practitioners must look at the new ways and implement the already identified ways of improving QOL, well-being, enhance hope and build resilience amongst cancer patients of each type.

The results have further indicated that emotion focused coping and problem focused coping total did not show any consistent correlation with these positive mental health indicators. Therefore, it is not about training the patients on either problem or emotion focused copy while looking at the ways of coping based intervention amongst cancer patients. Rather the specific emotion focused coping and problem focused coping interventions are required to be known for improving different indicator of positive mental health.For example hope and resilience can be enhanced in multiple ways as various ways of coping were found to be positively correlated. But distancing seems to be most important regarding QOL and health related well-being of cancer patients.

Appropriate strategies required for patients as per individual needs should be looked for and patient must learn that. Similarly it is very important to understand that „accepting responsibility" does not work for cancer patients. They might rather not like to hold them responsible for their disease as it reduced many aspects of QOL and health related well-being. Planful problem solving also affects different aspect of QOL and health related well-being differently. So this can also not be a generalized strategy for improving the positive mental health of cancer patients. However, much work is needed on this and research must be furthered. Distancing, in any case, has been recommended by earlier researchers in the west also.In the present Indian study also it has proven to be the best.

It is also concluded that one needs to look for specific intervention that is effective for a particular type of cancer. Ideographic approach since to be important.Results of PMR training are also extremely encouraging. It improved all indicators of mental health in all types of cancer taken in the study. This is simply a reflection on positivity created by PMR. Therefore, learning and regular use of Progressive muscle relaxation contributes to improvement in quality of life, well-being, hope and resilience. The result of phase II are all the more encouraging as all groups of all types of cancer patients were benefited by PMR on QOL, subjective well-being (FACT-G), hope, resilience, ways of coping, fatigue and hospital anxiety & depression. This can be recommended and can be integrated as a part of treatment. The method of PMR used in this study was simple and eight sets of muscles were involved. It took only 20 minutes in administration and can be administered by self after learning it appropriately for 4-5 sessions CD and other mode of recordings can also be used. On the basis obtained results it would not be an exaggeration to say that in patients with cancer, Progressive muscle relaxation should be integrated with chemotherapy to increase its efficiency, particularly because it is not easy to design „tailor made" intervention for different patients and different type of cancer as required and concluded on basis of results of part I.

The use of Progressive muscle relaxation, as a non-pharmacological measure, in cancer patients should be ensured.

Suggestions/ Recommendations

- Sample in the phase II of study was taken from a limited area (Rohtak and nearby areas). However, it could have been from a wider area for wider applicability and stronger generalizations. The study must be repeated at various places or with a larger representation of various areas of the nation.

- The result indicate that type of cancer is an important factor affecting the positive mental health, but hardly any studies have been conducted by taking different types of cancer. In view of the obtained differences in various types in this study, it is suggested that more studies should be conducted by considering different cancer types.

- Indian studies are also very limited in number. As the results of some of the past studies have shown that effects may vary in different nations, conducting more Indian studies bears high relevance.

- The research on ways of coping in India needs to be furthered.
- Short term and long term effect of PMR should be studied separately and qualitative analysis should also be done to understand how PMR influences the cancer patients.

- It is very important to sensitize the patients that they can live a good quality of life and enjoy good status of health related well-being even with cancerous body. It is all about their attitude particularly the distancing from the disease symptoms.

- In view of the observed deteriorated positive mental health among cancer patients, it is recommended to oncologists that the mental health enhancing interventions should be an integral part of the treatment package.

- It seems necessary to design and apply the hope improving interventions for the patients of cancer. This stands true at least for the Indian population.

- Also it is necessary to include the required interventions to raise QOL, subjective well-being, hope and resilience amongst the cancer patients as a part of treatment package.
- It is clear that various indicators of mental health are differently correlated and separate interventions may be required to enhance different indicators of positive mental health. Therefore, more studies need to be conducted to further the research.
- Though it has been suggested that type specific interventions should be designed, yet PMR has proven to be a generalized strategies. PMR has been found to enhance mental health of cancer patients irrespective of cancer types; so oncologists must include PMR in treatment.
- PMR should be accepted as an adjunct to cancer treatment.
- Government and hospital authorities should start employing counselors and psychotherapists to take care of the mental health of cancer patients.

Limitations

- The process of working in the hospital for data collection of phase II was completed and a relaxation room was prepared in the cancer ward of PGIMS Rohtak. But the environment in the hospital was not ideal and it was less congenial for giving PMR to the patients. The ward used to become noisy sometimes. Also many patients used to go home after chemotherapy and those seeking radiotherapy were not being admitted sometimes. This made data collection difficult in the hospital. Some of these were coming from the distant parts of the state and were relieved before completion of a month practice. This also involved lot of cooperation and commitment on the part of patients as they had to especially come for relaxation only. So the drop out was very high, as many times a patient would not be able to come either due to severity of symptoms or distances. Consequently the data could not be collected in the hospital. This not only delayed the collection and completion of data but also many patients had to be dropped out. The researcher could not rely on stage 3 and 4 patients only; 2nd stage was also included. The patients were then contacted from the OPDs in Rajiv Gandhi Cancer Hospital, Delhi.

- To tackle this, issue the patients were identified and PMR was given individually at their home. It not only took much longer a time for collection of data in phase II but PMR could also not be given in groups. Group PMR is sometimes more effective. However, this does not seem to have influenced the results. PMR in groups might have speeded up the process. It is also more motivating.
- Due to time limit, the frequency of people using different types of coping in different types of cancer could not be analyzed.
- All groups could not be completely matched on socio demographic variables in spite of our best efforts.
- Earlier it was planned that PMR would be given to the patients who would be distinctively low on mental health as assessed in phase one. But later on all of them could not be contacted and PMR was given to any patients who consented or were available. This also did not affect the results as pre-post differences were analyzed for testing the hypotheses, but the originally proposed design guidelines could not be met.
- Since allthe group results were analyzed separately, the comparative effectiveness of PMR on different groups could not be analyzed.
- Residual effect of PMR could not be studied due to time limitation.
- Researcher was unable to find the studies in which various types of cancer have been compared to understand how these differ from each other. So the results could not be compared with past studies regarding which type of cancer has been a worst or least hit on various variables studied i.e. QOL, FACT-G, hope, resilience. So more studies should be done in this area.

CPSIA information can be obtained
at www.ICGtesting.com
Printed in the USA
LVHW081815261122
734044LV00013B/510

9 783576 144705